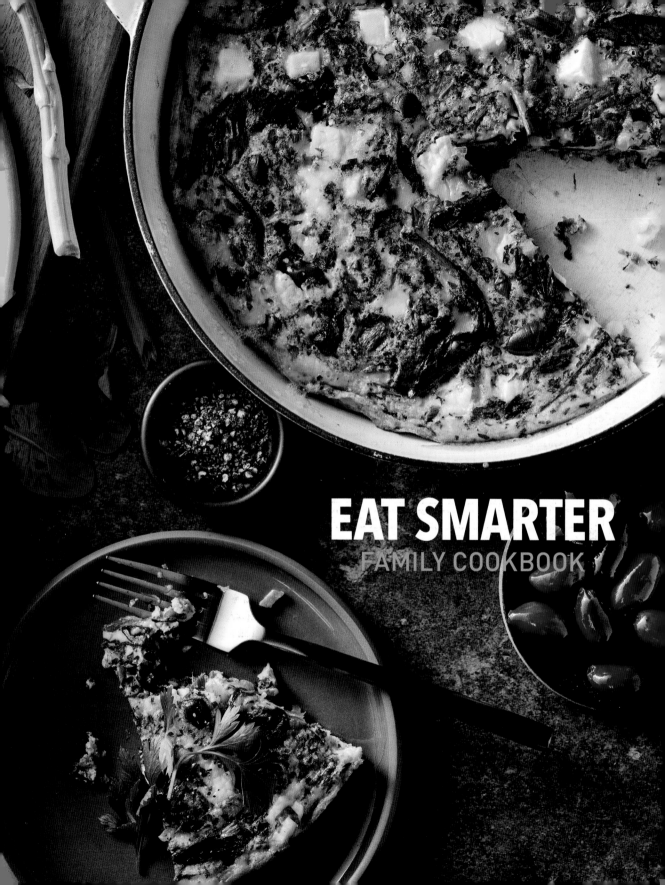

EAT SMARTER

FAMILY COOKBOOK

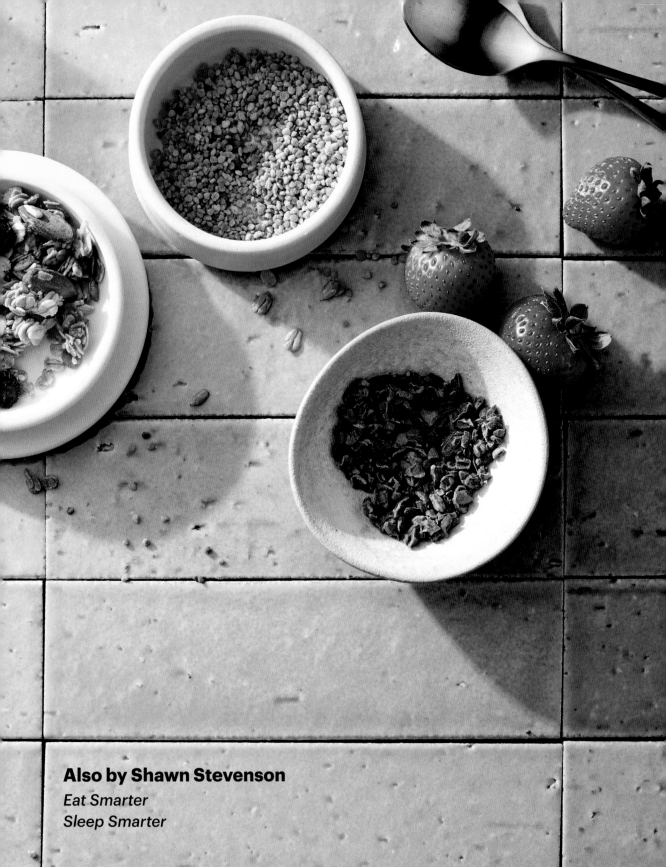

Also by Shawn Stevenson

Eat Smarter
Sleep Smarter

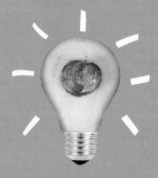

EAT SMARTER
FAMILY COOKBOOK

100 Delicious Recipes to Transform Your
Health, Happiness, & Connection

Shawn Stevenson

PHOTOGRAPHY BY EVA KOLENKO

LITTLE,
BROWN
SPARK

New York Boston London

Little, Brown Spark
Hachette Book Group
1290 Avenue of the Americas, New York, NY 10104
littlebrownspark.com

First Edition: October 2023

Little Brown Spark is an imprint of Little, Brown and Company, a division of Hachette Book Group, Inc. The Little, Brown Spark name and logo are trademarks of Hachette Book Group, Inc.

The publisher is not responsible for websites (or their content) that are not owned by the publisher.

The Hachette Speakers Bureau provides a wide range of authors for speaking events. To find out more, go to hachettespeakersbureau.com or email HachetteSpeakers@hbgusa.com.

Photography © Eva Kolenko
Book design by Laura Palese
Food styling by Carrie Purcell and Nicole Twohy

ISBN 978-0-316-45646-3
Library of Congress Control Number: 2023936319

10 9 8 7 6 5 4 3 2 1

TC

Printed in Canada

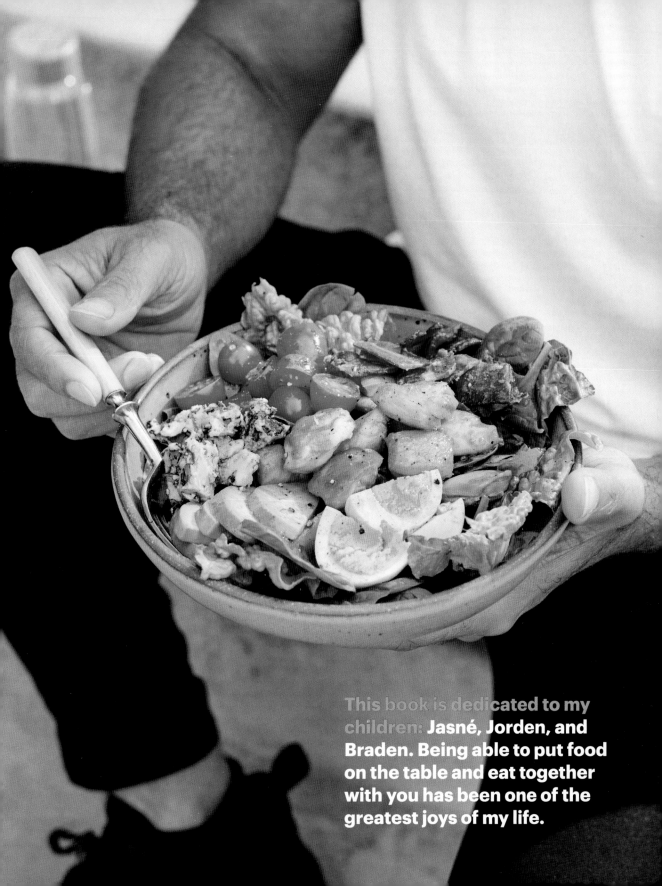

This book is dedicated to my children: **Jasné, Jorden, and Braden. Being able to put food on the table and eat together with you has been one of the greatest joys of my life.**

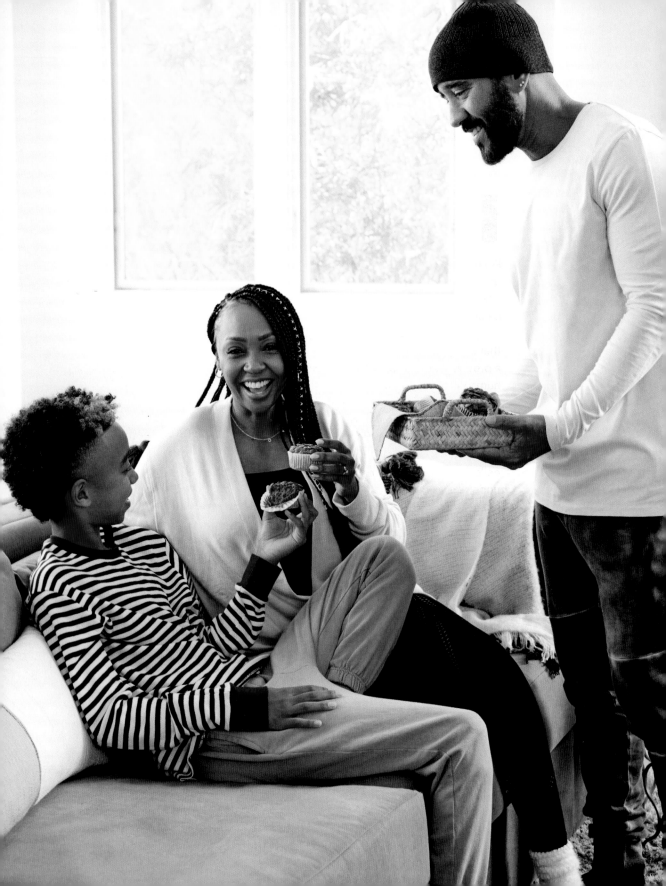

Introduction

I'm truly honored and grateful to be able to share this cookbook with you. One of the biggest lessons I've learned while working in the field of health and wellness the past twenty years is that food can be a powerful tool for happiness and healing, but it can also be a powerful weapon for degradation and disease.

Food is one of the most powerful entities in our universe—and I don't make that statement lightly. The food that we eat literally becomes a part of us. Through a process that's nothing short of miraculous, food is able to be transformed into human tissue. Every cell in your heart, your brain, your bones, and your belly is made from the food that you eat. Food is what makes us who we are. But in many ways, we've lost sight of this.

In my university biology classes, while learning about the wondrous world of our cells, my classmates and I were never taught that the quality and content of our cells would be determined by the food that we eat. There was a disconnect from understanding that our mitochondria were made from our meals, our nuclei were made from nutrients, and our membranes were made from our menu. In essence, we were given an assumption that these parts and processes "just happen." And this lack of awareness has filtered its way through every part of conventional medicine.

The highest levels of training in health care and medicine receive a staggeringly small amount of education in nutrition. Oftentimes, that education is superficial and positions food as just "fuel" or a means to avoid deficiencies. The dominant role that food plays in health is simply not understood. The average cardiologist, as brilliant and caring as they might be, has little conscious awareness that the organ they are treating is made from the food their patient has eaten. They're operating blind to the fact that the veins, arteries, and makeup of blood itself are all made from their patient's diet. Could this missing link in health care be the reason behind our epidemics of chronic diseases that have skyrocketed in recent decades? I believe that once we truly understand how much food matters, we will see a revolution in the health and well-being of our society.

Food Literally Saved My Life.

In my darkest days, food came to the rescue and helped me reshape my mind and body. At just 20 years old, I was diagnosed with an advanced arthritic condition of my spine. My bone density was so low that I broke my hip while running, and I was a few drive-thru menu items away from no longer recognizing myself in the mirror.

I was tip-toeing into obesity as stealthily as a ninja. My residual self-image was that of someone who's a fit athlete who could perform at any given moment. But my life circumstances were that of someone who was living with chronic pain, addicted to fast food, and gaining so much weight that my booty broke through the frame of my couch when I sat down one day. Did that experience help me realize that I needed to make some changes and get healthy? Well, in the words of Forrest Gump, "The only good thing about being wounded in the buttocks is the ice cream."

So more ice cream it was! But only the premium cheap stuff from Dairy Queen...added to my usual rotation of McDonald's, Burger King, Taco Bell, Popeye's Chicken, and Papa John's Pizza. I ate fast food 300-plus days of the year for several years. And when I wasn't eating fast food, you'd find me dining on a box of Velveeta Shells & Cheese (yes, the whole box was my meal), a family-sized can of beef ravioli, or one of many cartoon character–laden boxes of cereal. I was eating myself into an early grave, yet not one of my physicians asked me about my diet.

A massive meta-analysis published in *The Lancet* in 2019 titled "Health effects of dietary risks in 195 countries" examined the links between poor diet and the skyrocketing rates of chronic diseases in our world today. **The scientists determined that poor diet kills 11 *million* people around the world every year.** The researchers stated, "Our findings show that suboptimal diet is responsible for more deaths than any other risks globally...highlighting the urgent need for improving human diet across nations."[1]

Poor diet is responsible for more deaths than any other issue in the world. *Why is this not breaking news every day?* The situation is beyond dire. But the good news is that we know what the problem is, we understand the social systems that enabled this to happen, and we now have clinically proven strategies to turn this situation around.

It's important to know that we don't get to this level of disease and dysfunction from tripping and falling face-first into a box of Twinkies. There are coordinated efforts by processed food manufacturers, lobbyists, friendly government regulations that corroborate the processed food industry, and relentless marketing of low-quality foods—with an especially malicious aim at our children.

That's how Cap'n Crunch and Ronald McDonald got their hooks in me. I was young, impressionable, and my developing brain didn't stand a chance against the well-funded teams of food scientists who were formulating fake foods to make them irresistible. My childhood was filled to the brim with fake foods and their even faker mascots. I saw Toucan Sam on the television telling me to "follow your nose" to a box of Froot Loops, and that's just what I did. I didn't have any context to understand that he could be lying to me right through his rainbow-colored beak. And I was far from alone.

A report published in *Archives of Pediatrics and Adolescent Medicine* detailed an eye-opening study that tested if placing a cartoon character on the box of cereal influenced children's taste preferences. The children were asked to taste test what they believed to be different cereals and rate them on a five-point smiley face scale. Some of the cereal boxes had cartoon mascots, some did not. Even though the cereal was actually the same, kids consistently rated the taste of the cartoon-featured cereals better.[2]

Every day, processed food companies are manipulating our families biochemically *and* psychologically. By the time I made it to college, I was so inundated and addicted to chemical-laden processed foods that nearly every meal I ate was devoid of meaningful nutrition. And as a result, my health was rapidly falling apart.

Physician after physician told me that my condition was "incurable" and it was something that "just happens," which was very similar to the ideology that I picked up in my university education as well. But something just didn't add up. There was another principle that kept gnawing at me: the concept of *causality*.

Nothing in our identifiable reality "just happens." There are specific causes for the effects that we see and experience. We might not be able to consciously pinpoint what those causes are. But just because a well-meaning expert can't explain what the reason for the effects are, it doesn't mean that our circumstances are just a stroke of bad luck. After several years of pain and suffering, I finally asked myself a couple of important questions that changed everything:

"If my spine and bones are degenerating, what's causing the degeneration? What are my spine and bones actually made of?"

And since my attention had been solely focused on disease and I'd been outsourcing my health to others that entire time, it was like a switch was flipped on in my mind. I asked: "What can **I** do to feel better? What can **I** do to get healthier?"

By changing my perspective, I suddenly felt less like a victim and more like I had influence over my actions and outcomes. When I began asking better questions, it led me to better answers. Eventually, I realized that our bodies simply can't build our tissues correctly without being provided with the raw materials to do so. Our bodies are incredibly intelligent and resilient, and if forced to, they can do a patchwork job to try to hold our health together. But what if we provided our bodies with the essential nutrients required to build robust cellular structures? And what if we avoided the things that are proven to tear those cellular structures down?

Some of the critical nutrients needed to shore up my bone density went beyond the call for calcium I'd seen in commercials. Celebrities donning Steve Harvey–sized milk mustaches were telling me a tall glass of pasteurized, homogenized milk would give me strong bones. Yet no matter how much milk I was guzzling, I was feeling more like Mr. Glass than Mr. Incredible. By investigating what's really required for great bone density, I learned about dozens of other powerful nutrients that I rarely received on my drive-thru diet. Nutrients like vitamin D, vitamin K, magnesium, zinc, and amino acids like glycine were all noted in peer-reviewed studies to improve and support bone density. Even omega-3 fatty acids have been proven to contribute to bone mineral density. A study published in the peer-reviewed journal *PLoS One* found that the consumption of omega-3s can improve bone mineral density specifically in the hips and the lumbar spine—the two regions where my body just happened to be breaking down![3]

Omega-3s are some of the most delicate, most easily damaged compounds in nature. With the way that I was eating, it's not an exaggeration to say that I could easily go years at a time not getting in a viable source of omega-3s. But now that I knew what to target, I felt like there was a powerful momentum shift happening in my favor.

I could've easily become a natural pill popper and started gobbling up synthetic forms of all the nutrients I needed. And, actually, I tried that for a bit. I got a little bit better, but I also got a lot broker. Buying all of those supplements on my college student budget was not going to cut it. However, the process of figuring things out for myself led me to one of the most overlooked keys in all of health.

The nutrients needed to be *bioavailable*—that is, efficiently assimilated and utilized by my cells. In our haste to dominate and control nature (the central tenet in modern science), we have missed out on the fact that there's an underlying intelligence that animates all of life. **When you isolate things into parts, you negate the power of the whole.** A synthetic nutrient, though it may have the same chemical makeup, does not have the underlying intelligence or, even more tangibly speaking, the supporting elements and nutrient cofactors that magnify its resonance with our human cells.

Food isn't just food; it's information.

Take vitamin E, for example. This nutrient is important for healthy function of your cardiovascular system, cognitive performance, and even the health of your skin. Well, a study published in the *American Journal of Clinical Nutrition* determined that natural vitamin E has nearly *twice* the bioavailability of synthetic vitamin E. What about the fan favorite vitamin C? Renowned for its support of our immune systems, it's also important for improving our sleep quality, supporting cardiovascular health, and it's one of the most powerful antioxidants ever discovered. A study cited in the *Journal of Cardiology* put a vitamin C–dense berry up against a synthetic vitamin C supplement to see which one was more protective against a potent oxidative stressor like smoking. The study had twenty male smokers consume camu camu berries (one of the highest botanical sources of vitamin C) daily over the course of a one-week study and found that it led to significantly lowered oxidative stress and inflammatory biomarkers such as C-reactive protein. What's more, there were *no* changes in these markers in the group who received an ordinary synthetic vitamin C supplement. For the researchers, this indicated that the combination of other antioxidants from the berries had a more powerful antioxidant effect than synthetic vitamin C products alone.[4,5]

Food isn't just food; it's information. And real food has the intelligence and resonance with human cells to make all the difference in the world. Once I understood this, I began to focus on eating foods that were rich in the nutrients my body had been craving. These real, delicious, nutrient-dense foods began to transform my body from the inside out. Within a matter of days, my energy levels began to increase and I felt more motivated, optimistic, and capable. Within a matter of weeks, the pain I'd been experiencing for years began to fade away and I began to release the fear of moving my body. I didn't need pharmaceutical drugs to help me get around anymore, and the pain was no longer waking me up at night. And within a matter of months, I'd lost nearly 20 pounds, my skin was glowing, and my body was transforming in ways I couldn't have imagined.

Real food saved my life, and it ignited a fire in me to inspire and serve others. I began working as a trainer at my university gym, and after graduating I began teaching cutting-edge nutritional science to individuals and organizations all over the world. It's been surreal to see all that's transpired the past twenty years in

Friends, family, and food are going to be there to help guide you on your <u>mission</u>. And I'm going to show you how. You're about to <u>discover</u> some mind-blowing facts about food that will change your life <u>forever</u>.

this field. I've had the honor of working with organizations ranging from Google to ESPN. I've lectured everywhere from the neuroscience department at New York University to the cold climate and warm hearts of the students and faculty at Dalhousie University in Canada. There was a time when all of the speaking and traveling for my mission was frequently taking me away from my family. Nowadays, they're usually accompanying me on these adventures, and the mission of improving our society's wellness has become a family affair.

I believe that we can leave our world, and the health of our communities, better than we found it. But for that to happen, we have to find ways to innovate, to connect, and to empower. That's the reason that I started my show ten years ago, when podcasting wasn't, yet, a part of our popular lexicon. It was to provide the education that I wish I would've had access to when I was struggling to turn my health around. I know, firsthand, the power of awareness, access, and opportunity. And that's the passion I put into every episode and the thousands of hours that have been invested into uplifting every person I can. *The Model Health Show* has been the number one health podcast in the US many times over the years. But what makes that statement truly special is that it was created by someone who was led to believe that he was unhelpable; someone who believed that his conditions of pain, poverty, and despair were his destiny; someone who'd hit rock bottom and finally decided that it was a firm place to stand up.

I don't believe that there's anything particularly special about me. To me, we are all so beautiful, phenomenal, and capable that it's difficult to articulate. The rub is that we must each decide, as an individual, to unlock that beauty and capacity within us. We have to decide who we're going to be in this world and how we're going to serve. It takes a tremendous amount of courage to work on ourselves and decide to express more of our potential. But the good news is that we don't have to do it alone.

Friends, family, and food are going to be there to help guide you on your mission. And I'm going to show you how. You're about to discover some mind-blowing facts about food that will change your life forever. Plus, **this is change that you actually get to eat!** Within these pages are a plethora of amazing recipes deliciously designed with a specific purpose. The bridge that I crossed, going from the drive-thru diet that was promoting my illness, to real-food nutrition that was promoting my health and vitality, was much more fun and easier than most people realize. Having a family, there was no way we were going to go from eating the processed food in a value meal to serving my kids a sliver of romaine lettuce topped with a dropperful of hypoallergenic hummus. We would've had a revolt from the townspeople! Just picture the kids in your family coming at you with pitchforks—or any forks, for that matter. Neurosis and diet dogma are not necessary. Our number one objective is to make delicious meals we know and love while radically upgrading their ingredients. That's what transformed my health and the health of my family, and that's what I've had the honor of teaching countless others to do along the way.

The companion to the cookbook you are holding in your hands, *Eat Smarter: Use the Power of Food to Reboot Your Metabolism, Upgrade Your Brain, and Transform Your Life*, took off like a rocket when it was released. It was the number one new release of *all* books on Amazon, a *USA Today* national bestseller, a top 10 audiobook, and several other incredible accolades. But what most surprised me about this important "big idea" book that was dedicated to teaching people about metabolic health, cognitive health, emotional intelligence, and more, was how many readers were making and posting recipes from the book and sharing them with their friends and family online. Even with the paradigm-changing information in the book, it still boils down to making tasty meals and eating them. That's what inspired me to create this *Eat Smarter Family Cookbook*. So let's get started with the life-changing insights that will help you stack conditions in your favor!

Family Matters

CHAPTER ONE Eating smarter is about much more than preparing and eating delicious foods. It's about going beyond the plate to upgrade your environment so that healthy eating becomes *automatic*.

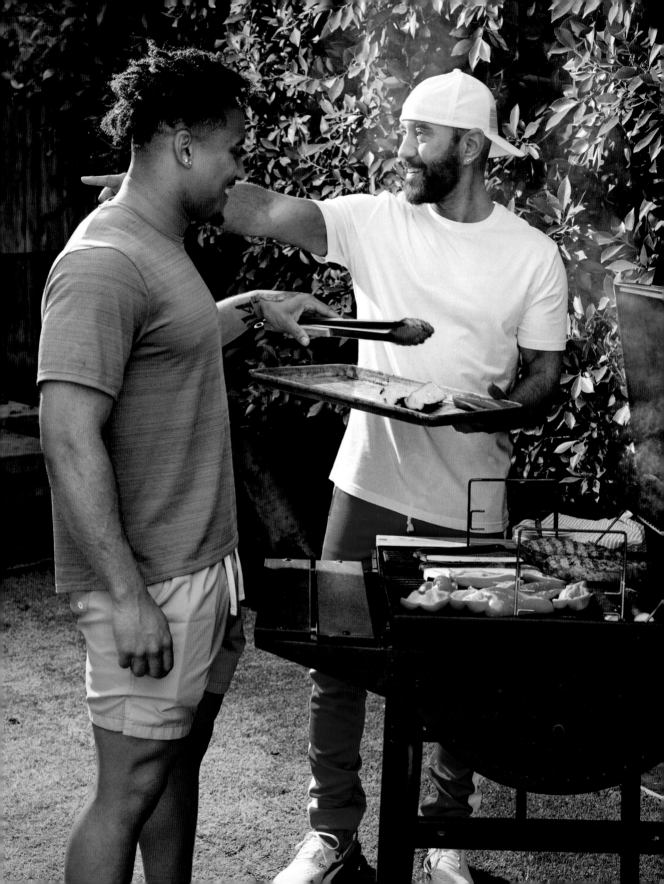

We might be under the illusion that we are making the choices of what we eat by our own free will. But the research clearly indicates that our environment and, more interestingly, *whom* we're eating with have a huge impact on our diet and health outcomes.

For thousands of years prior to our current generation, food centered around more than just the act of eating. Food was about family. Food was about sharing and cooperation. Food was about celebration and community.

We've quickly shifted from a species that prepared and ate food together for millennia to frequently eating in isolation with processed foods and mind-numbing media. What is the real impact of this shift in behavior? **Did eating together help protect human health in some way?**

Several studies have now demonstrated how much the simple act of eating as a family can influence the outcomes of our food choices. For instance, **researchers at Harvard University recently uncovered that people who consistently eat dinner with their families frequently consume more fruits and vegetables and less soda and processed foods.** Their data analysis also showed that increased frequency of family dinner was associated with higher intakes of several nutrients that support health and defend the body against diseases. Specifically, eating together as a family increased consumption of fiber, calcium, folate, iron, B vitamins, vitamin C, vitamin E; lowered glycemic load; and lowered the intake of trans fats.[1]

FACT: The conditions in which we eat have a profound impact on <u>what</u> we eat.

If we're constantly trying to target the food choices themselves, without addressing the environment and the family culture around eating, we are truly doing ourselves a disservice. Having a family ritual of eating meals together makes it *easier* to eat better things. The consistency in routine, the intentional meal planning, and the elimination of distractions are just some of the reasons this simple act can have such a huge impact.

Another study, cited in the *Journal of Nutrition Education and Behavior,* found that children who ate breakfast with their families at least four times a week were more likely to consume adequate amounts of nutrient-rich fruits and vegetables. The study went on to report that children whose TV was never or rarely on during family meals were significantly less likely to consume soda and chips. And children who consumed breakfast, lunch, *or* dinner with their family at least four days per week ate at least five servings of fruits and vegetables the vast majority of days each week.[2]

What's specifically interesting about this study is that it was incorporating data from minority children who generally lived within the construct of low-income communities. This shines a subtle but hopeful light that even if we don't yet have access to the best food options, creating and sustaining a new family ritual of eating together more often can dramatically improve the health outcomes of our families.

In the introduction to this cookbook, I shared how I grew up inundated with ultra-processed foods. Oftentimes, my family struggled to get by. There were times that we'd receive food from charities, we'd receive food from government assistance programs (unless you've had government cheese, you simply can't understand government cheese), and more often than not, my mom would have to make a dollar stretch further than your favorite yoga pose.

My parents did the best they could with what they had. But none of us understood how much the heavily processed foods we were eating every day was influencing our health outcomes. As a result, essentially everyone in my family and extended family had at least one chronic disease—obesity, heart disease, diabetes, asthma, eczema, and depression, to name a few.

We were literally surrounded by fast-food restaurants and liquor stores overflowing with heavily processed foods. The food was cheap, accessible, and artificially designed to tantalize our taste buds. But it wasn't just the external environment, or the food itself. It was our family culture around eating. It may sound unreal, but I can count on my two hands the number of times my family actually sat down and ate a meal together. We'd often eat at the same time, but it was more like a free-for-all. Everybody would grab something and eat wherever we could sit, often in front of the television, and often with the trappings being ultra-processed foods.

With these pieces of data, it can become easy to place blame on our caregivers for our personal habits. But that's not what this is about. I simply can't blame my parents for my eating behavior. It was a cultural phenomenon.

But here's where our power truly resides. We are not just products of our environment, we are *creators* of our environment. Once we become aware of how our environment is shaping our choices, we can make simple yet powerful shifts in our environment to make healthier choices more accessible. Again, the process starts with awareness.

For example, despite our economic status, had we known that simply eating together as a family more often could provide an added defense against illness and improve our health outcomes, we could've taken advantage of it. Now that I have this information within my grasp, I can use it to stack conditions in my family's favor and help spread this empowering information to every family possible.

This education is needed more than ever. Along with the steady decline in family meals, there's been a steady increase in our society's consumption of heavily processed foods. Today, according to data published in the *BMJ*, **nearly 60 percent of the average American's diet consists of ultra-processed foods.** This is a shocking statistic, when only a fraction of that amount was common just a few decades ago. And the worst impact is happening to our kids.[3]

A new study published in the *Journal of the American Medical Association (JAMA)* analyzed the trends in ultra-processed food consumption by young people between the ages of 2 and 19 over the past two decades. The study found that from 1999 to 2018, the average American youth's ultra-processed food consumption went from an already staggering 61.4 percent of their diet to an even more alarming 67 percent! In association with this growing trend, childhood obesity has tripled in the last thirty years. We cannot stand idly by and allow this crisis to continue. It's up to us, as parents, to make changes at home that can filter their way out to the community at large.[4,5,6]

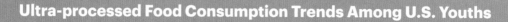

Ultra-processed Food Consumption Trends Among U.S. Youths

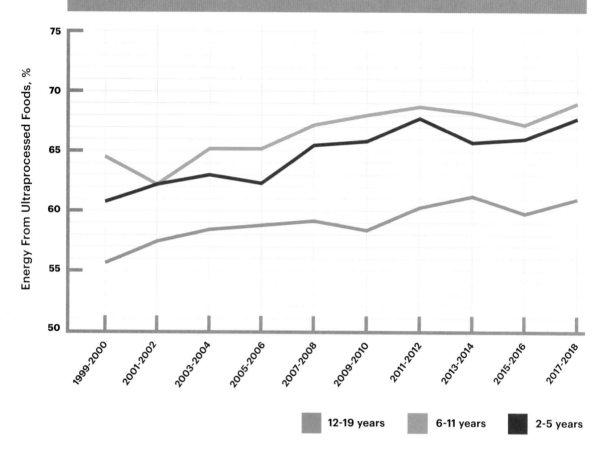

According to data published in *JAMA Network* and the journal *Pediatrics*, children and adolescents are at vulnerable stages for the development of environment-fostered obesity. The researchers uncovered that eating together as a family more often provides an added layer of protection against obesity and more. The data revealed that **children and young adults who share family meals three or more times per week are more likely to be in a healthy weight range and**

have healthier eating habits than those who share fewer than three family meals together. Additionally, and incredibly important, these children were far less likely to engage in disordered eating. Just three family meals per week is the minimum bar to set to provide an additional layer of real health insurance.[7,8]

Eating together isn't just great for kids, it's amazing for parents, too. A study cited in the journal *Family and Consumer Sciences* disclosed that sitting down to a family meal helped working parents reduce the tension and strain from long hours at the office. The researchers found that even if test subjects had major stress at work, if they could make it home in time to eat dinner with their family, their employee morale stayed high. However, as work increasingly interfered with the ability to eat dinner with their family, levels of dissatisfaction at work began to creep up. It's still not widely understood how devastating excessive stress can be to our well-being. According to data published in *JAMA Internal Medicine*, **upwards of 80 percent of all physician visits today are for stress-related illnesses.** Stress is exacerbated when we're not eating well and not getting enough healthy social connection. Eating dinner with people you love is a surprising buffer against that stress that more people need to know about.[9,10]

Despite all of the psychological and biological benefits of eating together seen in studies, according to researchers at Harvard University today **only about 30 percent of families manage to eat together regularly.** Again, the cultural norm of eating together as a family has steadily declined in recent decades, while our consumption of technology and ultra-processed foods has steadily gone up.[11]

A startling truth is that our devices can divide us. Used intentionally and responsibly, our technological innovations can help us to connect in many ways. But as the research indicates, jacking into the matrix through our screens can have us immersed (and even addicted) to a virtual world and missing out on the real world—and real people—right around us.

We all love the experience of getting together to watch a movie or a big game with food, friends, and family. This can be a wonderful event to take part in. Yet when meals in front of screens becomes the daily norm, as it is for many families, social and eating dysfunction is likely not far behind.

Television programming has been programming our families for decades. America literally invented the concept of the "TV dinner" back in the 1950s. The ads showed happy families huddled up around the television with their freshly reheated frozen dinner trays. The ads would say things like "Ready in minutes…No work and no dishes!" That's like straight-up sexy talk to parents in an increasingly fast-paced world. The catch was, this act of dissociation leads to overlooked stress in other ways. Let's take a look at the field of epigenetics to understand why.

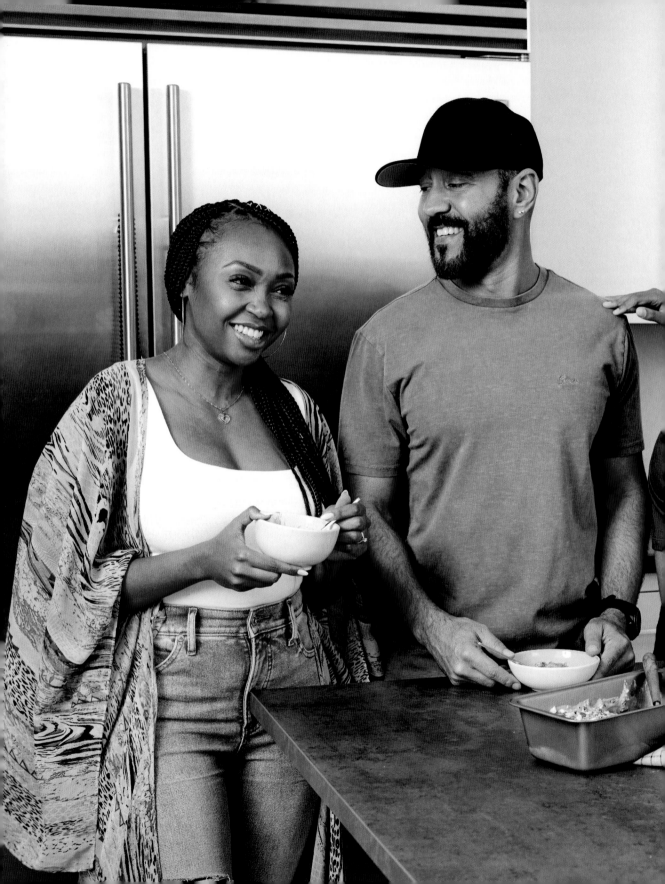

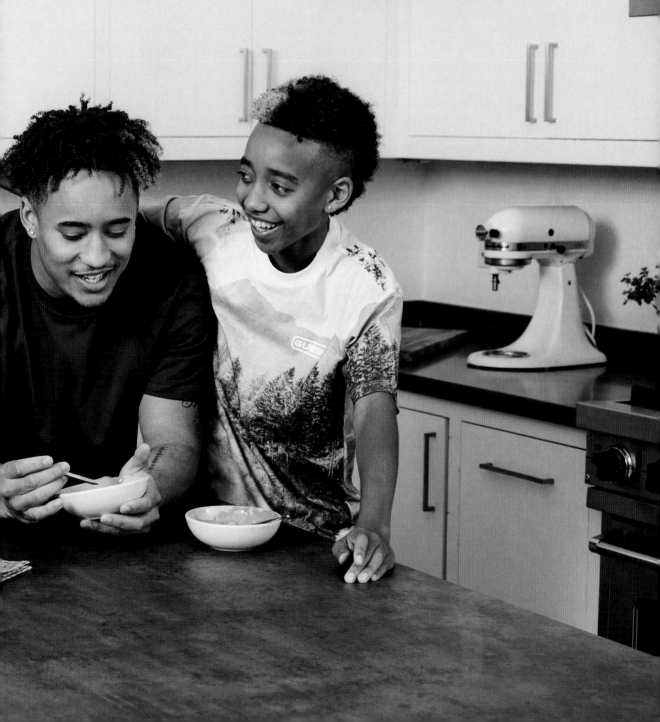

We are not just products of our environment, we are creators of our environment.

Your genes expect you to connect.

I first learned about epigenetics during a lecture from renowned cell biologist Dr. Bruce Lipton many years ago. The prefix *epi* means "above," and epigenetics is the study of our cellular function *above* genetic control. In college, I was taught about health through the lens of the "central dogma." This was the belief that your genetic information flows only in one direction, from DNA to RNA to protein. There is no room for change. Your genes control everything about you. And there's nothing you can do about it. The central dogma is like Sho'nuff from the movie *The Last Dragon*, swearing that he's "the master." But in reality, when you truly understand epigenetics, that's when you realize you have the power to access "the glow."

I was led to believe that I was simply the victim of some bad genetic cards, and that my health problems were something that "just happens." But in reality, I had elicited the function of several epigenetic factors that were causing my DNA to "print out" lower-quality copies of me.

Yes, we all have genetic predispositions for certain conditions, but as a recent study published by researchers at UC Berkeley concluded, **only a tiny fraction of diseases are caused by true genetic defects.** The report, titled "Genetic Factors Are Not the Major Causes of Chronic Diseases" elucidates several epigenetic environmental and lifestyle factors that actually promote disease expression— things like smoking, deficiency in critical nutrients like omega-3s, and the consumption of trans fats from heavily processed foods. But one of the fastest growing epigenetic factors being studied is interpersonal human relationships in the real world.[12]

A collaborative analysis from scientists at Stanford University and the University of Illinois states: "Genes in the brain are malleable, turning on or off in response to internal and external cues...[and] *social signals* can have a profound effect on when and how genes function." Social animals (not just humans) *require* healthy social interactions for optimal function and maintenance of DNA. This is why our relationships are emerging as one of the most potent epigenetic controllers influencing our health.[13,14]

A meta-analysis of 148 studies tracking over 300,000 participants uncovered that **adults with strong social ties have a 50 percent boost in longevity versus individuals who don't**. I want to take a moment to appreciate how profound this really is. According to the scientists at Brigham Young University who compiled this data, healthy relationships can contribute up to a 50 percent reduction in risk of death from *all* causes. In fact, strong social relationships were more indicative of longevity than exercising or beating obesity.[15]

Now, that's not to say that exercise and having a healthy body composition are not incredibly important. But it highlights that there's a lot more to health and longevity than the standardized things we're programmed to think about. Community and connection are things that are encoded in our DNA. Our genes *expect* us to have strong bonds to other humans. It's how we evolved...it's how we made it to this point as a species. Yet today, in many ways, we are more isolated than at any other time in history.

On the surface, it can look as though we're more connected than ever. We may have hundreds or even thousands of friends through online social networks. We have Skype, Zoom, FaceTime, and so much more to see people face-to-face virtually. We have access to countless online groups and so many other virtual ways to connect. But something is missing...

A report from the National Academies of Sciences, Engineering, and Medicine demonstrates that in the US, more than one out of every three adults aged 45 and older feels lonely. And research utilizing the UCLA Loneliness Scale revealed that loneliness scores are highest in people between the ages of 18 to 22 years old. **The study demonstrated that well over half of our population feels lonely.** And the rise in social media use has paradoxically increased loneliness, with 73 percent of heavy social media users ranking high in loneliness scores, as compared with 52 percent of light social media users ranking high in loneliness. Neither fact is good. And it's having a serious impact on our health.[16,17]

The report succinctly detailed that:

- Social isolation significantly increases a person's risk of premature death from all causes.

- Social isolation is associated with about a 50 percent increased risk of dementia, currently the sixth leading cause of death in America.

- Having poor social relationships, as characterized by social isolation or loneliness, is linked to a 29 percent increased risk of heart disease and a 32 percent increased risk of stroke.

- Loneliness is strongly associated with higher rates of depression, anxiety, and suicide.

Again, these results don't "just happen." Our real-world relationships are crucial epigenetic controllers that determine our health outcomes. On the empowering side, this is another factor emerging from studies on healthy centenarians (people who live to be 100 years old or more). **There are wide-ranging diet and exercise habits from centenarian to centenarian, but community and social connection consistently stands out as a definitive factor for longevity.**

Yes, technology can ignite and support relationships. But there's something vital about connection in the real world that simply cannot be replaced. Let's use this powerful science as a call to action for our little ones, elder ones, and everyone in between. Part of healing our health struggles is being more intentional about coming together with friends and family and eating together more often. **The dinner table can truly act as a unifier.** Sharing a meal is the perfect opportunity to catch up, talk, and connect with those who matter most. It's cool that we have our hustle muscles flexing big time in our world today (we've got some work to do!), but it's also absolutely critical to decompress. And doing that along with good food and family can transform our reality.

Here are some tips to start utilizing to radically up-level your nutrition, your health, and your relationships.

No. 1 Schedule It!

Today, it's easier than ever to have random things invade your good intentions. Rather than leaving things up to chance, block off specific times each week that are sacred for your family. The very best data we have shows that three meals per week together with your family is the minimum bar to see some profound improvements in nutrition, mental health, and overall health outcomes. More is fine, but three is the minimum bar to set.

This can be breakfast, lunch, dinner, or even a combination of different meals. For example, you could block off Monday, Wednesday, and Thursday for family dinners. Or family dinners can be scheduled for Tuesday and Thursday, plus a family brunch on Sunday. Or, say you work in the evenings, and family breakfast together Monday through Friday works best. There are many ways to slice and dice this. But the most important thing is that it complements your lifestyle and family goals in the most graceful way possible.

Remember, it's essential to schedule it! Put it on your calendar and set a reminder. It's a vital step towards making it real.

No. 2 Make It a Phone-Free Zone

This is one of the most important things you can do to be more present and make the most of your family meal times. The science is very clear on this. Devices *will* divide you. If you want to connect and reap the health benefits we've covered, it's a must to set up a phone-free parameter.

A plethora of studies demonstrate how the active use of smartphones reduces our awareness of the external environment, distracts our focus, and contributes to diminished performance when multitasking. When you are scrolling social media while simultaneously talking to a friend, you are definitely not 100 percent present with your friend. That's obvious. But what's not so obvious is that the mere presence of your phone, whether you're on it or not, has been proven to reduce your mental capacity. Researchers at the University of Texas at Austin conducted fascinating studies to test a variety of cognitive processes while test subjects had their phone facedown on the table next to them, versus having their phone in their pocket or backpack, or having it in another room entirely. Having the phone within their field of vision led to *significant* reductions in their cognitive capacity. (The researchers surmised that the presence of their phones reduced their mental energy or caused more "brain drain.") Having their phone in their pocket or backpack near them caused slight reductions in cognitive capacity as well. But in both instances, the participants subjectively didn't think that having their phone near them affected them at all. They were severely wrong. They believed, as most of us do, that as long as they're not on it, it's not a distraction.[18]

The reality is that we have a very strong cognitive association with our phones and what they give us access to. According to another study published in the journal *Social Psychology*, even the sight of *someone else's phone* distracts our attention. The researchers detailed how the mere sight of a smartphone turns up our awareness of the "broader social community" we can access through that device. This attention-robbing experience is largely unconscious. But it's just the tip of the iceberg of the growing body of science revealing how our devices are impacting our brains.[19]

The bottom line: Accessing the benefits of eating together with your family means not bringing your digital teleportation device to the table with you. Make a pact with your family to leave the smartphones in another room, tuck them away out of arm's reach, or implement another creative way to keep your phones from trespassing on your family time.

No. 3 Embrace the Adjustment (and Be Kind to Yourself)

When making changes to your family's routine, there's naturally going to be an adjustment period. Some families find out about the benefits and protective elements of eating together as a family and immediately find a rhythm that works and enjoy the process right off the bat. Some families—particularly if eating together has been rare and devices have been the usual meal companions—have a little more turbulence when making family meals a new part of the family culture. No matter what boat you're in, you can get the ship sailing to more connection and better family health. Remember, you are the captain of the ship. You can fly by the seat of your pants like Captain Jack Sparrow, or you can intentionally guide your crew to the destination you want to arrive at.

The first step is clarity. What is the end result you want? What is your north star? Communicate that with your family. Be a benevolent leader and say, "This is what we're doing as a family,...this is the direction we're going,...and here are the reasons why."

For example, let's say your end result is having family dinner together three nights per week. Communicate your mission statement with your family: "We are going to make it a power-packed family tradition to have dinner together Sunday, Monday, and Wednesday each week. This is something we're all going to make sacred, and support each other on. We're going to do this to ensure that our family is able to connect because I love you so much. And I want to make sure that we're all creating healthy habits that you'll be able to pass down for generations to come."

Whatever the goal you have is, whatever the reasons might be, a little communication can go a long way.

Again, some families hop right on board and enjoy the new open waters. Other families might have some questions about the voyage, while other families might have a member or two who feel like they'd rather walk the plank.

One of the simplest ways to get your kids on board is to get them *involved*. Ask them for input on what an awesome family dinner would look like. Ask them questions about what could make it more fun and rewarding for them. Maybe they'd love family dinner to be outside one of those nights each week, whether it's a patio, a blanket in the backyard, or a picnic table at a nearby park. There are so many flavors of what an outdoor meal can look like. Maybe they'd like to have a special seating arrangement, a special premeal ritual, or a special dessert. There are so many ways to help them be involved in the process. You'll likely find that when you

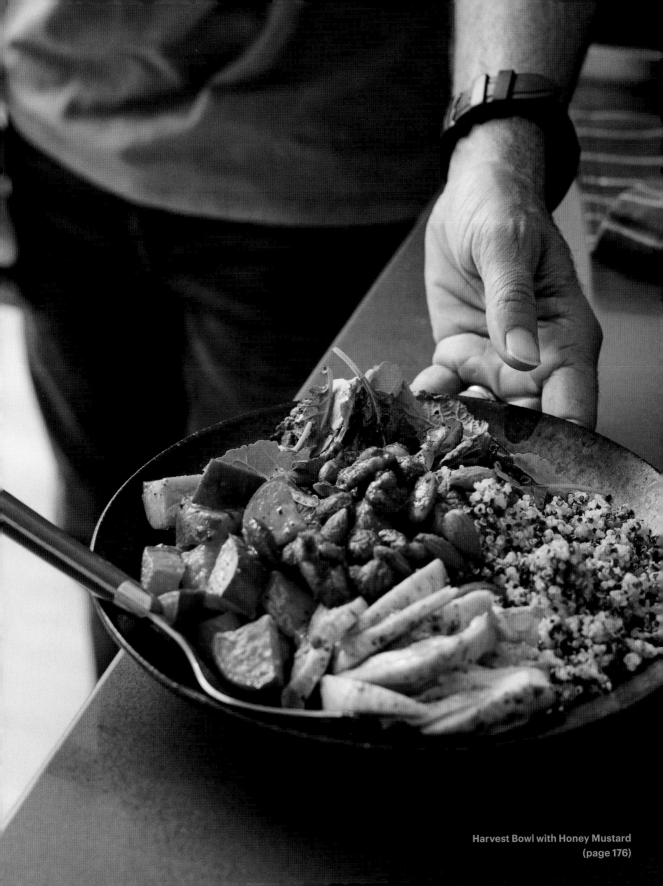

Harvest Bowl with Honey Mustard
(page 176)

give them specific choices (A or B), they're more willing to oblige, and even more happy with the outcome.

Be kind and patient with yourself. But also be firm in your intention. Everything will not always go according to plan, but you are more than capable of navigating choppy waters. For instance, the kids might not be thrilled about getting off their screens for family meals initially, especially if the family culture has previously been screen-heavy. But those cognitive patterns that make their devices so alluring can be tamped down and changed. You have to understand that their little brains can get addicted just like ours do. As a leader, you have the ability to know your family members' personalities and what motivates them. Use your benevolent influence to guide them in the desired direction. And definitely take advantage of the next tip!

No. 4 Put Some Icing on the Family Time Cake

One of the most common mistakes people make when taking on a new habit change is taking away what they're used to and replacing it with something of far less value. If you're going to suddenly take away your favorite rich, full-fat chocolate ice cream and replace it with a sugar-free, fat-free, dairy-free, gluten-free, pleasure-free (I might as well lick a chocolate-colored ice cube) alternative, you're probably not going to be happy with that switch. And you're probably going to have a vendetta for the person who told you it was a great idea to do that in the first place.

When making a habit change, replace old habits with things that feel as though they're of equal or greater value. The key word here is *feel*. Because this is all just neurochemistry that we produce in our own bodies based on how we perceive things. If you're taking away my screen with entertaining cartoons, maybe provide me with some great entertainment in the real world to counter that. Maybe it's a debate about the top 10 cartoons of all time over dinner. (True story: We've had some "passionate" debates about the best Marvel movies several times.) Maybe it's playing some of your kids' favorite songs. Maybe it's a post-dinner rap battle. Maybe it's a spiciest hot sauce challenge or a weird food challenge. There are countless ways to make family dinners memorable and blow passive entertainment from devices out of the water. Be playful, experiment, and double down on what works best.

No. 5 Stick to the Script When Ordering In

Things happen! Maybe you intended on making a wonderful home-cooked meal for one of your scheduled family meal days. But there was a curveball at work, or your kid's sports practice, or the day just got away from you. There's no need to throw in the towel and relent to ordering food and then you and your family eating parked in front of a device. Simply get your takeout or delivery and sit down and eat together as intended. Just because you got the curveball of not being able to cook, doesn't mean that you can't successfully hit the ball and still make the experience special.

The more that you allow unexpected circumstances to get in the way of family meals, the more you'll find that unexpected circumstances keep coming up. Stick to the script as much as possible so that *habit becomes necessity* and *family meals become family culture.*

No. 6 Extended Family and Friends Count, Too!

The power of eating together with people you care about is not merely reserved for your nuclear family. Having meals with friends and extended family will pour on the same benefits. As we've discussed, more people are eating alone today than ever before. A peer-reviewed study published in *Nutrition Journal* in 2018 found that people who eat alone tend to have poorer diet quality and lower intake of essential nutrients than people who eat with others. There is a proven remedy to this situation. But because our eating behaviors are largely unconscious, the average person simply doesn't know that eating with others more often can provide a buffer against some of the most common poor eating outcomes.[20]

If someone lives alone, having just a few meals a week with friends or family can make a world of difference. Make it a must. Be the catalyst to schedule meals each week with friends or extended family members. Help bring people together, be intentional, and continue to unlock the many benefits of eating smarter.

Transform Your Kitchen Culture

CHAPTER TWO   Culture is defined as the set of attitudes, values, beliefs, and behaviors shared by a group of people and communicated from one generation to the next. We can see the outward results of different cultures— how different cultures dress, how they eat, how they communicate, etc.—but we don't often think about the underlying attitudes, values, and beliefs that make those visible outcomes possible.

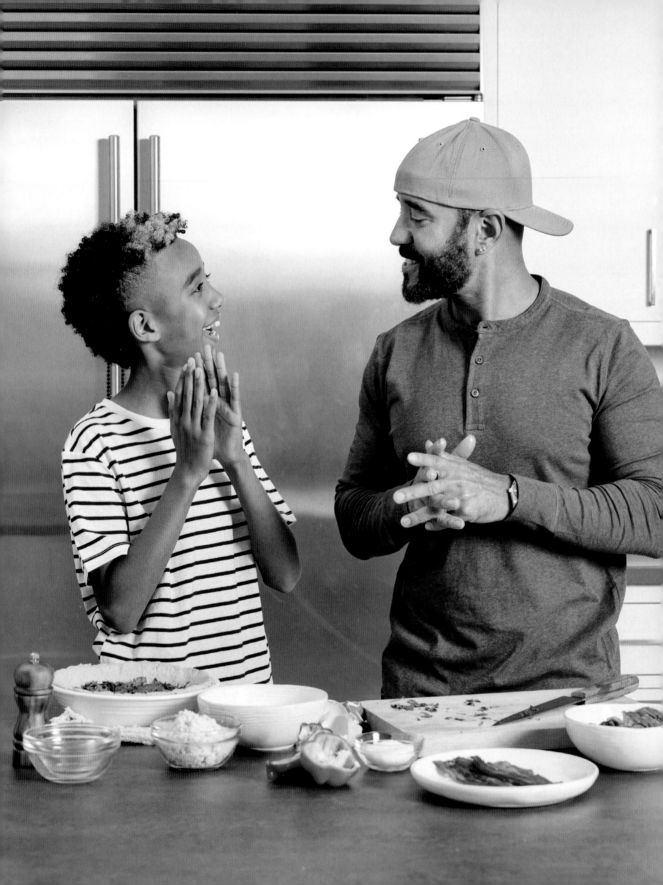

The culture we exist in is sort of like an invisible guidance system that directs us towards certain things and away from others. For example, there are still cultures that require physical activity from their members in order to gather or hunt to have food to eat. The cultural belief is that "if you don't move, you die." The culture directs them towards movement and skills that invoke cooperation and natural food selection. And the culture blocks them from the awareness that 7-Eleven exists where they can easily throw their spear through a hot dog or honeybun.

People born into some cultures today know the sound of a fountain soda dispenser far better than they know the sounds of nature. When I was a kid, I had no idea that the can of Planters Cheez Balls my mom bought weren't "good for me," let alone what those sad, orange, air-filled little balls were made of. To us, they were simply viewed as food. To another culture, they could be viewed as poison, or as a handy alternative to Styrofoam packing peanuts.

It's critical to understand that our cultural influences are largely *unconscious*. We don't choose the culture we're born into. We simply begin adapting to the culture we're raised within whether we realize it or not. Humans are born as base

Our society is obsessed with trying to change <u>behaviors</u> without addressing the underlying <u>culture</u> that the behavior is stemming from.

models with our factory settings; then the culture we're raised in determines the accessories we're equipped with. Some of us end up fully loaded with knowledge and habits of exercise, good nutrition, and healthy relationships. Others, like myself, are fully loaded with high fructose corn syrup and a chip on their shoulder that makes them 1) want to fight the world and 2) dip that chip into Cheez Whiz.

When you change the culture, you automatically change the attitudes, values, beliefs, and behaviors of the people within it. Unfortunately, our society is obsessed with trying to change behaviors without addressing the underlying culture that the behavior is stemming from. It's very much like superficially treating the symptom of a disease without addressing the underlying *cause* of the disease. You can try to treat the symptom or behavior all day. But if you don't address and change the root cause, the symptom or behavior will inevitably come roaring back.

We are going to target healthy habit change at its core by intentionally and intelligently adjusting the culture our habits spring from. Though there are larger cultural containers that we exist within (country, state, community, etc.), the most practical and impactful level of cultural change is the one within our own household. When we adjust this, miracles happen that have a tendency to spread far outside of our front doors. This is because wherever you go, you take your culture with you. Transforming your family culture is the first step in transforming your world.

Eat Smarter

Defend Your Family Against Cultural Contagions

You are the one endowed with the power to lead your family's superhero team. And with any good superhero team, there's going to be a menacing villain. When it comes to our family's health, that villain is processed food companies. Much like Professor X, they have proven abilities to control our minds and bodies. But they use their power for profits and care little about the Carnage they leave in their wake.

According to data published in *The BMJ* (as noted in Chapter One), nearly 60 percent of the average American's diet consists of ultra-processed foods. And the statistics are even worse for our children, *who are growing up in an ultra-processed food-laden culture*, with approximately 67 percent of the average child's diet in America being made of ultra-processed foods. For the food companies, from manufacturers all the way to retailers, business is booming!

US grocery stores (where the bulk of our ultra-processed foods are being copped) are pulling in *hundreds of billions of dollars annually*. And when I say this is where ultra-processed foods are mainly being dealt from, I'm not exaggerating. A recent study published in the *American Journal of Clinical Nutrition* found that approximately 61 percent of the foods sold by US grocery stores is ultra-processed foods. That number just so happens to reflect the amount of heavily processed foods the average person is eating. But the grocery stores are just the middlemen. Processed food companies are the Kingpin driving the system.[1]

A not-so-fun-fact is that in terms of revenue, the largest privately held corporation in the entire US is a processed food manufacturer. Cargill, along with three other food companies, control approximately 70 percent of the global agricultural market. It doesn't take Superman's X-ray vision to see this is a problem. If you control the food, you can control the people. And what are their primary agricultural products that are being used to flood our communities with ultra-processed foods? Sugar, pesticide-laden grains, and highly refined vegetable oils.[2]

Sweeteners

SCARY CHOICE	SUFFICIENT CHOICE	SMARTER CHOICE
Artificial sweeteners	Organic cane sugar	Raw honey
Conventional sugar	Organic coconut sugar	Stevia
Corn syrup	Dried fruit	Monk fruit
High fructose corn syrup	Organic grade B maple syrup	

Shift the culture around sweeteners

Humans have had a relationship with sweetness for tens of thousands of years, at least. Sweetness, once exclusively found in whole, real-food sources, signified a dense source of energy and valuable micronutrients that came packaged in natural foods. Remember, food isn't just food, it's *information*. Food communicates its nutritive qualities in a language we call flavor. There's a phenomenon called post-ingestive feedback where your brain creates biochemical "tags" to remember which nutrients (and in what amounts) are attached to which flavors.

The problem is not this immaculate natural system that's been refined over hundreds of thousands of years. The problem is that we're now swimming in fake foods that have been artificially crafted by brilliant, Dr. Doom-level food scientists to muddy up the waters of this sophisticated communication and make us crave a dangerous abundance of sweet things. Again, it's not our inherent desire for sweetness; it's the manipulation of our biology and the sheer amount of sugar we're surrounded by.

In the 1700s, the average westerner was consuming 4 to 6 pounds of sugar each year. Today, the average American consumes more than *10 times* that amount! Data published in the peer-reviewed journal *Advances in Nutrition* states that **the average American now consumes 80 pounds of *added* sugar every year.** To be clear, this is the amount of sugar added to foods on top of the already existing sugar and/or carbohydrates in the food products. Combining the existing sugar in a typical highly refined grain–based diet with the added sugars, the average American is consuming well over 100 pounds of sugar each year. It's staggering.[3]

Not so surprisingly, nearly 130 million Americans now have type 2 diabetes or prediabetes. And a recent study published in the peer-reviewed journal *Metabolic Syndrome and Related Disorders* determined that **only 12 percent of American adults are metabolically healthy.** Something is severely wrong. And it's going to take families of Avengers to step up and put an end to this.[4]

There are three simple steps to creating a force field that defends your family against the heaviest impact of sugar. Again, this is not about neurosis and eliminating sugar completely; that's simply not logical or necessary for the average family today to radically improve their health outcomes. This is about shifting the family culture, a few steps at a time, to make healthier choices automatic.

Step 1

Reduce the amount of prepackaged processed foods that you buy.

A huge percentage of the average family's sugar intake comes from the added sugars in ultra-processed foods. Conventional cookies, cakes, candy, crackers, chips, snack bars, and the like typically make up the lion's share of sugar intake from food, especially for kids. By slashing the amount of prepackaged foods you bring into your family's superhero headquarters, and instead, making some of the simple, delicious grab-and-go treats from the *Eat Smarter Family Cookbook*, you'll be outfitting your family with a suit of armor that even Iron Man would marvel at.

Step 2

Upgrade your sweeteners—and keep low-quality sweeteners out of your home.

A symbol of modern life is our abundance of options. And true to form, these options can be helpful or harmful, depending on how we associate with them. When it comes to food selection, there are *smarter* options, *sufficient* options, and options that are outright *scary* that should have your Spidey-sense tingling whenever they're around. Conventional sugar is devoid of any nutrition at all, a quick contributor to high blood glucose, and one of the most pesticide- and herbicide-laden commodity cash crops.

One of the many herbicides used in sugar production is the highly controversial glyphosate. Data published in the journal *Interdisciplinary Toxicology* details how glyphosate can increase the risk of everything from cancer to celiac disease to infertility. The most alarming thing is that this study was published almost ten years ago! Numerous peer-reviewed studies have come out since on the clear detrimental impact of glyphosate. Even the World Health Organization has classified glyphosate as a group 2A carcinogen, denoted as a *probable* carcinogen to humans. Why in the world is this still used heavily in our food supply? That conversation is for another day, but you'd better believe it has a lot to do with a word that starts with "mo" and ends with "ney." The good news is that we don't have to sit around and wait for food manufacturers to put ethics over profits. We can, right now, start reducing the amount of prepackaged processed foods we buy, and upgrade the quality of the sweeteners we use when the occasional recipe calls for it.[5,6]

Step 3

Distance your family from refined sugar–filled drinks.

The fastest method of flooding our system with sugar and causing metabolic dysfunction is through the consumption of *liquid* sugar, which is highlighted in a study published in the *Journal of Nutritional Biochemistry*. The researchers asserted that the consumption of highly concentrated liquid fructose (like what's found in soda) leads to the development of leptin resistance in the brain and the development of excess belly fat. Leptin is our body's primary satiety hormone. Drinking highly refined sugar–filled beverages leads to the one-two punch of 1) quickly creating more body fat while 2) making us want to consume more.[7,8,9]

In recent decades, beverage companies have been doubling down on sweetness as our society has been doubling, tripling, and quadrupling down on chronic diseases. Most citizens are not truly aware of the shocking amount of sugar contained in a single bottle of soda. For instance, a 20-ounce bottle of Coca-Cola is pouring 65g (about 16 teaspoons!) of sugar into your system. While my personal favorite growing up, 20 ounces of 100 percent pure orange juice, is not far behind with a whopping 56g (14 teaspoons!) of sugar going into your tank. It doesn't

Beverages

SCARY CHOICE	SUFFICIENT CHOICE	SMARTER CHOICE
Soda	Kombucha	Water (sparkling or flat)
Pasturized fruit juice	Coconut or water kefir	Low sugar kombucha
High fructose corn syrup	Fresh-pressed vegetable+fruit juices (be mindful of the sugar content)	Low sugar coconut or water kefir
Artificial colors or flavors	Fresh coconut water	Organic teas and coffee
Conventional pesticide/ herbicide-laden teas and coffee	Naturally sweetened carbonated drinks (great recommendations in the bonus resource guide!)	

matter much that it may have some vitamins in it. That amount of sugar is going to hyperstimulate insulin, damage leptin, and derange the communication between your brain and your body.

Because of their liquid form, these inordinate amounts of sugar hit your bloodstream with the speed of The Flash. The superior approach is to treat liquid sugar like kryptonite and keep it out of your family's home. Relegate it to special events or outings, or better yet, upgrade the go-to beverages for your superhero team overall. Remember, you have the power to decide the culture you create from here on out. Whether you have the Infinity Gauntlet or not, with the snap of your fingers you can change your family's destiny and the destiny of generations to come.

An Important Note on Artificial Sweeteners

One of the steps promoted to reduce our sugar intake is to simply switch to artificial sweeteners. Essentially, the belief is: "You'll get the sweet taste but none of the metabolic problems caused by sugar." Of course, this marketing is coming straight from processed food manufacturers. The artificial sweetener market is a multibillion dollar industry, driven primarily by an even bigger multibillion dollar soft drink industry. Going to a soda company for a healthy beverage is like going to Batman for a hug. It's not going to happen. The fact that soda companies are so sweet on artificial sweeteners should immediately raise some red flags. Despite the obvious conflicts of interest from known abusers of public health (the soda industry), and despite the growing body of evidence against artificial sweeteners, there are some folks still reaching out for artificial sweeteners like Thor reaching out for his hammer.

A recent study conducted by researchers at the Boston University School of Medicine and published in the peer-reviewed journal *Stroke* uncovered a surprising link between drinking diet soda and two debilitating health issues. The study found that people who drink one or more diet sodas daily are almost three times more likely to have a stroke and develop dementia than people who have less than one diet soda per day or don't drink them at all. Now, just to be clear, this is a strong correlation, not causation. But the researchers did an excellent job taking into account adjustments for age, sex, education (for the analysis of dementia), caloric intake, diet quality, physical activity, and smoking. This should be enough to at least raise a few eyebrows as to why there could be a connection with artificial sweeteners and the brain. Let's take a look at one of the most obvious reasons why.[10]

Artificial sweeteners actually do their work by tricking your brain. The taste receptors send messages to your brain that you're consuming something sweet. It would usually mean that your brain should expect some calories to accompany the sweetness but (surprise!) that's not the case. With the sweet taste coming in, and your body's primal programming to handle sweetness a certain way (through releasing insulin), it would be unwise to think we can fool our body's intelligence that easily. And a study from scientists at the Washington University School of Medicine confirms just that.

A recent clinical trial involving seventeen obese test subjects who did not regularly consume artificial sweeteners found that the artificial sweetener sucralose elevated their blood sugar levels by 14 percent and insulin levels by 20 percent on average! Artificial sweeteners can pretend that they're a superhero, but rest assured they're Loki in disguise, ready to take control of your brain and your hormones.[11]

An additional study, published in *Advances in Nutrition*, found that sucralose alters the microbiome in a way that promotes inflammation in animals. It also showed that mice given another popular artificial sweetener, saccharin, had increased expression of inflammation in their livers, which the researchers attributed to altered gut bacteria. Some experts rightfully point to the high doses of artificial sweeteners given in many animal studies. But the negative health alterations in this study were with 0.3mg of saccharin/mL, a dose equivalent to the FDA-approved acceptable daily intake for humans.[12,13,14]

As you can gather, there are a few concerns with both human and animal studies when it comes to artificial sweeteners. The biggest challenge today is that these topics tend to become so divisive. Sometimes, if we see something that goes against our beliefs, especially if that thing is working for us, we have a tendency to "shut off" or immediately reject information that goes against our perspective. Instead, we should strive to keep an open and curious mind and do what's best for ourselves and our families—and give ourselves permission to change over time if we feel good about it. If someone chooses to utilize an artificial sweetener in the context of an overall healthy diet, that can absolutely be an effective formula for them. Yes, because artificial sweeteners are a synthetic, newly invented substance solely designed to trick our brains and taste buds, they get an express pass into the *scary* category. But this is about progress, not perfection. This is about enjoying the process. This is about doing what's best for you right now and making changes towards less and less artificial stuff over time.

Use Your Superhero Brain When It Comes to Grains

In addition to sugar, the other category of foods that are keeping our communities' blood sugar levels in constant chaos is conventional grains. Though they are denoted separately on product labels, carbohydrates break down into sugar (glucose) in our blood. So when you combine our grain-heavy diet with the ungodly amount of sugars in our diet, you have a *Civil War* taking place within your metabolism that will break your body down from the inside out.

In my university nutritional science class, I was told how important "whole grains" were and how they should be the basis of our diet. So when attempting to improve my health, I went all in on whole grain everything. And, of course, the ringleader in whole grain marketing was "whole wheat." The first thing to note is that the type of wheat proliferating on store shelves today is not the amber waves of grain that our ancestors dined on. Wheat naturally evolved over thousands of years, but only to a modest degree. However, in the last couple of decades the makeup of wheat has been changed *dramatically* under the influence of agricultural scientists. Wheat strains have been hybridized and genetically manipulated to make them resistant to changes in environmental conditions and resistant to pathogens, and (most importantly for food manufacturers) to increase the speed of growth and yield per acre. This manipulation has essentially resulted in a food that the human microbiome has never seen before. And in recent years, we're seeing the results of it with growing numbers of people with celiac disease and gluten-related sensitivities. It's a real thing that's largely related to less-than-real wheat.

Gluten, one of the proteins in wheat, has emerged as a Green Goblin, flying in with inflammatory bombs and wreaking havoc. A recent study published in the peer-reviewed journal *BMC Biochemistry* revealed some shocking new data. In the study, the researchers found that digested gluten could block the ability for leptin to bind to leptin receptors. It was a dose-dependent response, as well. The more gluten present, the more leptin was blocked. In fact, the amount of gluten eaten in a typical meal of bread or pasta was found to reduce leptin binding by up to fifty percent![15]

Gluten has been portrayed in the role of the evil villain in nutrition for many years now. But I don't want you to get your crumbs in a bunch thinking that gluten-containing foods are off the menu. Indeed, to play it safe for many folks, it might be a good idea to be careful in teaming up with gluten, especially if you're dealing with insulin resistance, leptin resistance, or any inflammation-related problems. Data published in the journal *Nutrients* demonstrated that gluten prompts the

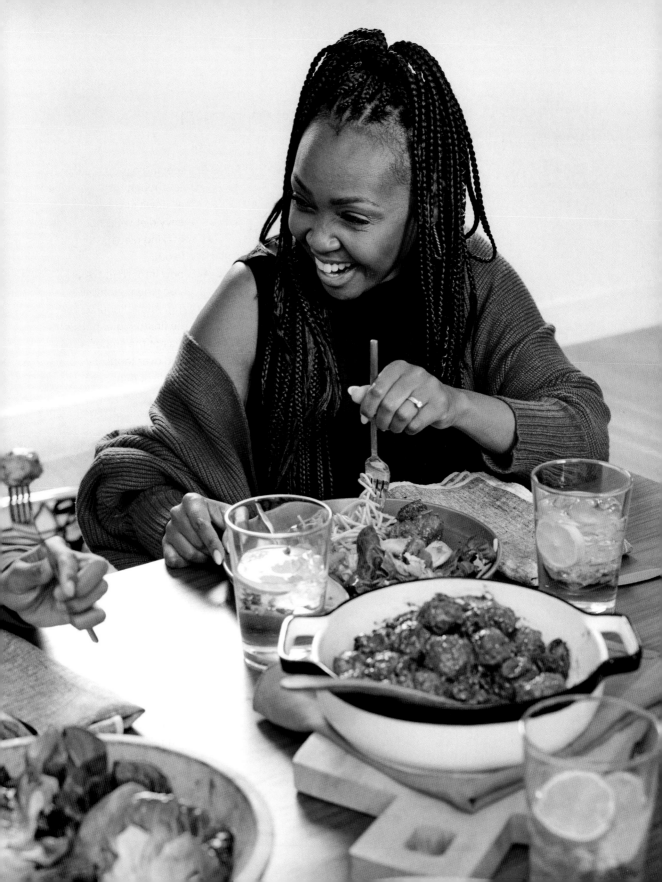

The vast <u>majority</u> of recipes in the *Eat Smarter Family Cookbook* are <u>gluten-free/grain-free.</u>

release of a protein called zonulin that increases the permeability of the gut lining, whether you are gluten sensitive or not. Dysfunction of the tight junctions that make up your gut lining is a key contributor to systemic inflammation. But as with most things, there are multiple perspectives to consider. Even the researchers in the study noted that the way the gluten was prepared/cooked made a difference in its effects on leptin. Still, the potentially bigger issue with wheat and other grains is the way they're grown and processed. If you upgrade the quality and avoid the following culprit, having occasional grains on the menu will not be a problem for most families.[16]

We touched on the heinous effects of glyphosate in the discussion around sugar. But according to the Environmental Working Group (EWG), wheat, oats, corn, and other bread/cereal grains are, by far, the largest source of glyphosate consumption for the average American today. Again, the World Health Organization has classified glyphosate as a group 2A carcinogen (probable cancer-causing agent for humans). Keep in mind, it's just one of *many* pesticides, herbicides, rodenticides, etc. used to grow the grain products that millions of unsuspecting people dine on every day.

The EWG published data affirming glyphosate contamination in 80 to 90 percent of popular wheat-based products. Another study on a wide range of popular breakfast cereals, oatmeals, and snack bars found glyphosate contamination in all of them. This included a variety of Cheerios, Quaker Oatmeal, and Quaker Chewy Granola Bars. The highest level of glyphosate found by the lab was 2,837 ppb (parts per billion) in Quaker Oatmeal Squares breakfast cereal, which

Grains

SCARY CHOICE	SUFFICIENT CHOICE	SMARTER CHOICE
Sprayed with pesticides and herbicides	Organic	Fermented (like sourdough)
GMO	GMO-free	Sprouted
High fructose corn syrup		
Artificial colors or flavors		
Made with conventional vegetable oils		

is nearly eighteen times higher than EWG's children's health benchmark. This was my absolute favorite cereal when I met my wife about nineteen years ago. She'll tell you that I'd have a couple of bowls every day because I believed it was a healthier option than the "kids cereal." Yet the sugar/carbohydrate content was identical and the things not on the label (the abhorrent amount of pesticides and herbicides) are waging *Secret Wars* on our communities.[17,18]

A couple of simple, quick steps to take when it comes to grain-based products are to 1) make it a mandate to go organic to avoid nefarious pesticides and herbicides and 2) go for sprouted and/or fermented products whenever you can, to increase the bioavailability of essential nutrients and reduce the presence of antinutrients. The vast majority of recipes in the *Eat Smarter Family Cookbook* are gluten-free/grain-free. But whenever grain-based ingredients are included, we follow that credo. A recent study published in *JAMA Internal Medicine* found that eating organic foods free from pesticides and herbicides led to a significant reduction in the risk of cancer for the nearly 70,000 test subjects who were analyzed. This is another change in the family kitchen culture that will stack conditions in your favor.[19]

Get Your Family's Oil Changed

Dietary fats are absolutely critical to human health and functionality. Fats are required as building blocks to make trillions of our cells and they're also utilized as metabolic fuel to run processes in our bodies. Being that fats are used to make our tissues *and* fuel our metabolism, the quality of fats we consume is of the utmost importance.

The fats we've eaten as humans for thousands of years have largely been swapped out within a single century. Contrary to popular belief, we are eating much less of the animal-based saturated fats that we evolved eating as a species, yet for some strange reason, our epidemics of obesity and disease have continued to climb even higher.

We've gone from the majority of our dietary fats being minimally processed animal and plant fats to today, where approximately 80 percent of the fat calories in the average American's diet is from heavily processed "vegetable oil."[20,21]

I put vegetable oil in quotes because its deceptive marketing label can evoke beliefs that it's healthy and smart to eat, or that it's even made from actual vegetables. But the truth is, the name "vegetable oil" is a misnomer. It's not made from vegetables at all. It's largely made from industrial seed oils, soybean oil, and a whole lot of synthetic chemicals. Learning how vegetable oil is made is something you have to see to believe. That's why I have a couple of videos for you to feast your eyes on in the bonus resource guide for the *Eat Smarter Family Cookbook* at eatsmartercookbook.com/bonus—you'll get to see firsthand how these seeds oils are processed at extremely high temperatures, scoured with chemical solvents, bleached, and then deodorized before it's promoted to be fit for human consumption. Even well-meaning experts still beating the drum of vegetable oil's safety can at least acknowledge that this conglomeration of oils is high in polyunsaturated fats that are highly unstable and sensitive to heat damage. Damaging these sensitive oils automatically increases their oxidative and inflammatory potentials in our bodies. They can try to change reality like the Scarlet Witch, but even they have to admit that vegetable oils fit firmly in the category of ultra-processed foods. To say these oils are safe or healthy is to ignore what they truly are.

More and more science is being published to affirm these facts. For instance, a meta-analysis published in the journal *BMJ: Open Heart* found that these vegetable oils can be a major culprit behind organ failure, cardiac arrest, and even sudden death. And to just give you a whiff of their volatility, research published in the journal *Inhalation Toxicology* found that even inhaling the smell of them while

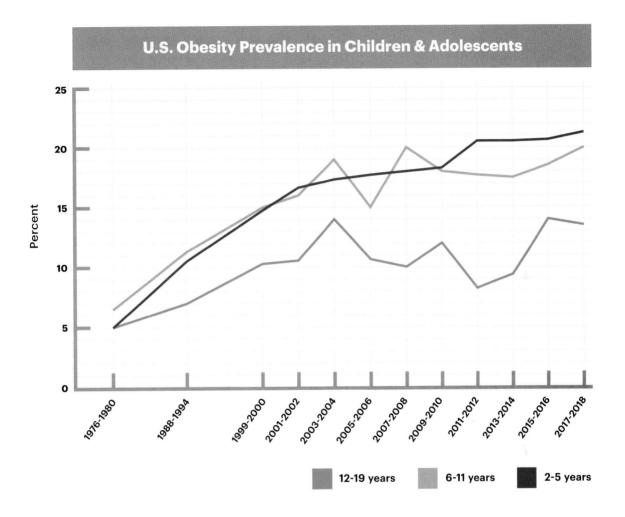

U.S. Obesity Prevalence in Children & Adolescents

Legend: 12-19 years | 6-11 years | 2-5 years

cooking can damage your DNA. The biggest offender, as noted in the journal *Environmental Science and Pollution Research International*, was the inflammatory fan favorite canola oil (aka rapeseed oil), coming in with the highest level of polycyclic aromatic hydrocarbons emitted into the room during cooking. Polycyclic aromatic hydrocarbons are implicated in everything from cancer to autoimmune diseases, but, hey, if we're encouraged to eat toxic foods, we might as well inhale their toxic smells in the process, too.[22,23,24]

To add injury to a *Deadpool*-degreed insult, recent research conducted by scientists at UC Riverside determined that soybean oil not only leads to obesity and diabetes, but could also affect neurological conditions like autism, Alzheimer's disease, anxiety, and depression. On top of the growing number of human studies, their animal study published in the journal *Endocrinology*, found that soybean oil negatively alters gene expression in the brain. These alterations were notable for increasing inflammation, disrupting insulin signaling, and more. And what can easily be overlooked in this study is that soybean oil was put up against an oil that's been utilized by humans for nearly 4,000 years, and this oil had none of the negative effects in the study that soybean oil did. That oil was coconut oil. Unfortunately, ultra-processed oils like soybean oils have been framed as healthy largely due to their lower ratio of saturated fats, while oils that undergo simple, time-tested extraction (without chemical additives and extreme heat) have been under attack. It was as if coconut oil was suddenly a mutant, and industry-backed scientists tried to make the saturated fat found in low-quality processed foods synonymous with the natural fatty acid profile in coconut oil. They are not the same. In fact, you'll discover some of the remarkable benefits of coconut oil and other time-tested fats that have been treasured by humans for millennia coming up in Chapter Three. For now, use these charts as a guide for your family's fats and oils. And use these additional food charts as a helpful ally along your mission to eat smarter.[25,26]

Cooking Oils

SCARY CHOICE	SUFFICIENT CHOICE	SMARTER CHOICE
Canola oil	Avocado oil	Organic avocado oil
Corn oil	Butter	Grass-fed butter
Soybean oil	Coconut oil	Organic coconut oil
Other "vegetable" oils	Extra virgin olive oil	Organic extra virgin olive oil
	Ghee	Grass-fed ghee

Beef

SCARY CHOICE	SUFFICIENT CHOICE	SMARTER CHOICE
Factory-farmed	Organic	Grass-fed/grass-finished
Grain-fed	Grass-fed/grain-finished	
Non-organic feed		
Heavily processed feed with artificial ingredients		

Poultry

SCARY CHOICE	SUFFICIENT CHOICE	SMARTER CHOICE
Factory-farmed	Organic	Pastured
Non-organic feed	Free-range	
Heavily processed feed with artificial ingredients		

Fish

SCARY CHOICE	SUFFICIENT CHOICE	SMARTER CHOICE
Farm-rasied (with non-organic feed)	Organic farm-raised	Wild-caught
Artificial color and perservatives		Low mercury
High mercury		

Eggs

SCARY CHOICE	SUFFICIENT CHOICE	SMARTER CHOICE
Factory-farmed	Organic	Pastured
Non-organic feed	Free-range	
Heavily processed feed with artificial ingredients		

Dairy

SCARY CHOICE	SUFFICIENT CHOICE	SMARTER CHOICE
Factory-farmed	Organic	Grass-fed
Grain-fed	Pasteurized/non-homogenized	Raw (from farms with high quality control)
Non-organic feed		
Heavily processed feed with artificial ingredients		

Spices

SCARY CHOICE	SUFFICIENT CHOICE	SMARTER CHOICE
Chemical flavor enhancers (like MSG)	No chemical additives	Organic
Synthetic preservatives	No synthetic preservatives	Freshly picked or packaged
Conventional salt	Higher quality salts (Celtic, sea salt, etc.)	

Family Snacks

SCARY CHOICE	SUFFICIENT CHOICE	SMARTER CHOICE
Sprayed with pesticides and herbicides	Made with higher quality oils (extra virgin olive oil, avocado oil, etc.)	Higher in protein
GMO	Non-GMO	Organic
High fructose corn syrup	No artificial ingredients	
Artificial colors, flavors, or preservatives	Low sugar content	
Made with conventional vegetable oils		
High sugar content		

Condiments

SCARY CHOICE	SUFFICIENT CHOICE	SMARTER CHOICE
Vegetable oil-based	Made with higher quality oils (extra virgin olive oil, avocado oil, etc.)	Organic
High fructose corn syrup	No artificial ingredients	
Artificial colors or flavors	Low sugar content	

Smarter Grocery Shopping

Another important aspect of up-leveling our families' culture around food is upgrading the way we shop for food. Here are a few key tips to add to your superhero utility belt.

No. 1 Watch Out for Healthwashing

Processed food manufacturers have stayed a few steps ahead of even health-conscious buyers by using trendy, health-affirming terms to make their products appear healthier and more nutrient-dense than they really are. For instance, there are marketing labels like:

- **Low Fat**
- **Made with Whole Grain Oats**
- **Naturally flavored**
- **Can help lower cholesterol**

Each of these labels has been slapped on boxes of a sugar-filled, ultra-processed, herbicide-laden breakfast cereal! This is the actual marketing used for Honey Nut Cheerios. And I know these healthwashing terms manipulate people, because they manipulated me. When I was trying to turn my health around in college, I saw these labels and thought this cereal was really going to help improve my health. In reality, it's a box of processed crap that's so far removed from anything natural that there's nothing "Cheeri" about it. The newest healthwashing label on this same popular cereal box is that it's "Gluten Free." Whether someone is truly gluten sensitive or not, this label denotes an added layer of benefit to it. But more than anything, it distracts from what the cereal really is: an ultra-processed junk food promoted by a googly-eyed bee with a dysfunctional stinger.

Sure, some of these healthwashing terms can also be applied to minimally processed real-food products. But more often than not, real food doesn't need to tell you that it's real food. Other healthwashing terms to be on the lookout for are:

- **All Natural**
- **Sugar-Free**
- **Fat-Free**
- **Fortified**
- **Enriched**
- **Made with real _____ (any healthy ingredient can be added to a recipe of unhealthy ingredients to make it look good)**

No. 2   Take Advantage of Sales

One of the things I learned to do while grocery shopping on a tight budget was to take advantage of sales and price cuts. Because of the way our food economy is currently constructed, it sometimes can be more expensive to buy higher-quality foods in conventional settings. So I kept my eye out for the sale items when I went to the grocery store each week. If strawberries were on sale, I'd stock up. I'd have some as one of my snacks for the week, maybe add some to a summer salad, and I could easily freeze the rest. The same thing went for the meat section of the store. If ground beef was on sale, we'd have a couple of meals featuring ground beef that week, plus I'd buy extra to pack away in the freezer. This method always saved me money when the month was over. Plus it helped encourage diversity in what I was buying since different things would be on sale at different times.

No. 3   Get Your Food Closer to the Source

So many incredible farmers' markets, CSAs, and food delivery sources have emerged due to the demands of more families who are dedicated to eating healthfully. Even while living in Ferguson, Missouri, I discovered that there was a weekly farmers' market just minutes from my house. It had been going on for years, but since I wasn't attuned to it—and didn't take the chance to look one up—I simply didn't know it existed. I saved money, got fresher food, and it was a wonderful experience to take my family whenever I went.

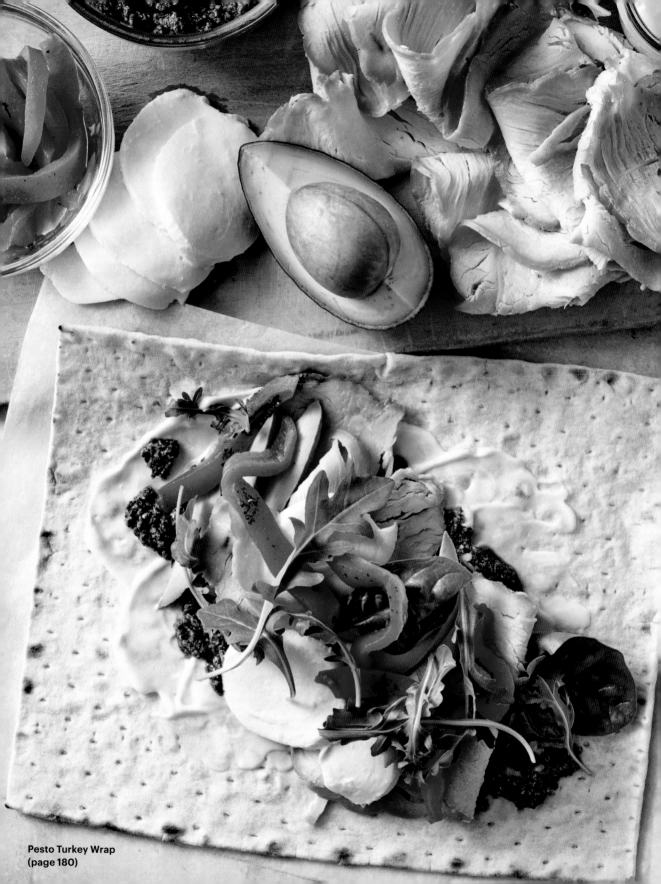

**Pesto Turkey Wrap
(page 180)**

In addition to farmers' markets and CSAs, there are some remarkable companies delivering the very best food in the world right to our doorsteps. Companies dedicated to regenerative farming, eliminating the use of toxic chemicals, and supporting the financial well-being of families by taking out excessive retail markups. You'll find a list of my favorite companies and links to learn all about them in the bonus resource guide at eatsmartercookbook.com/bonus. I encourage you to do your homework!

No. 4 Save Funds by Saving Food

Food waste is a huge problem in the US. Currently, we waste about 40 percent of the food we grow, contributing to the nearly 3 trillion dollars in global food waste annually! We've all done it, optimistically shopping: "Ah, let me grab another box of spring mix so that I can promptly throw it away in a few days." We can have the best of intentions, but our methods of keeping food fresh doesn't typically match that optimism. Here are a few simple tips to keep your food fresher longer and save funds by saving your food:

- Buy frozen, and/or buy fresh and freeze more often (this applies to everything from produce to meat).

- If you love to use fresh herbs like thyme, dill, parsley, and more, simply snip their ends and put them in a bit of water when you get home from the grocery store. Much like you do with a bouquet of flowers, that's how you want to treat your beautiful herbs. They'll often last one to two weeks longer this way.

- If you've ever had the non-pleasure of throwing away your salad greens just a few days after buying them due to wilting, do this simple step and that will be a thing of the past: Simply put a paper towel or two into your box of salad mix and it can extend its shelf life by several days. Today, there are even special veggie bags and freshness-extending paper products that you can use as well. A step that takes an additional minute can save your greens and save you money.

- Beef, poultry, and other meat should be kept in its original packaging if you're eating it within two to three days. If two days have gone by and you're not sure you'll get to it (regardless of your good intentions), simply play it smart by sticking it in a resealable bag and popping it in your freezer. You can always thaw it to use it whenever you're ready. **Better to thaw than to never use it at all.**

- Wash your berries in water and with a small splash of vinegar, then dry them well, before refrigerating them to help keep them fresh. Also, storing berries in specially designed berry containers, which you can buy once and use hundreds of times, is another simple way to extend your berries' life span.

- An avocado can be more of a choosey lover than just about any other food. One moment it's unripe and unfriendly; the next moment it looks like it's had one too many drinks and got into a bar fight trying to defend your honor. Avocado, I love you, but you need to be more balanced. Just before—or right when—your avocado becomes ripe, if you're not ready to eat it simply place it in the refrigerator to radically slow down its ripening.

These simple tips will help keep your food fresher longer. Plus, there are more tips in the bonus resource guide.

Now it's time to get into the kitchen, itself!

Smarter Cooking Tips

It's not just what we cook, but *how* we cook that can make all the difference in the world. Once you have great food in your hands, here are a few important tips to make the most of it.

No. 1 Use Nontoxic Cookware

One of the most impactful changes you can make in your kitchen is to swap out the toxic cookware that could be undermining your family's health. For decades, conventional nonstick cookware was used by millions of families every day under the assumption that it was safe. Conventional nonstick cookware is coated with a material called polytetrafluoroethylene (PTFE), commonly known as Teflon. It wasn't until just a short while back, in 2013, that one of the most nefarious compounds in Teflon cookware was finally removed. A chemical called perfluorooctanoic acid (PFOA) was shown repeatedly in peer-reviewed studies to contribute to higher rates of infertility, liver disease, and a variety of cancers. For instance, a study published in the *Journal of the National Cancer Institute* concluded that PFOA is a strong renal carcinogen with risk increasing in tandem with levels of exposure.[27]

The deflection point for years is that this only happens when Teflon pans are heated at high temperatures for long periods of time. The truth is, those variables change depending upon which dish someone is cooking. That should've never given PFOA a free pass. And more recently, data cited in the journal *Environmental Science and Pollution Research International* stated that even at normal temperatures, "PTFE-coated cookware releases various gases and chemicals that present mild to severe toxicity." They might have taken PFOA out, but it's clearly not the only concern with this toxic cookware.[28]

To upgrade your cookware, use these instead:

- **Stainless steel.** Stainless steel is time tested, incredibly durable, and relatively inexpensive. Stainless-steel pots and pans are great for sautéing and browning food. And stainless-steel baking pans are easy and dependable for popping a variety of foods in the oven. A stainless steel–based pressure cooker is a good option as well. Stainless-steel cookware is scratch resistant, long-lasting, and a staple for any healthy kitchen.

- **Cast-iron cookware.** When a cast-iron pan is seasoned properly, it makes a great upgrade for nonstick cooking purposes. It's perfect for high-heat cooking, and can easily go from stovetop cooking to being placed in the oven. If cared for, a cast-iron pan can last for generations. There's a simple, step-by-step video to show you how to properly season your cast-iron pan in the bonus resource guide at eatsmartercookbook.com/bonus.

- **Ceramic nonstick pans.** Ceramic nonstick pans have a familiar look and feel to conventional nonstick pans—but without the inherent toxicity. You can find ceramic frying pans and sauté pans that are PTFE- and PFOA-free, easy to clean, and with an occasional smidge of oil, wonderful for nonstick cooking purposes.

It's not just <u>what</u> we cook, but *how* we cook that can make all the difference in the world.

- **Glass baking pans.** This is another essential for healthy cooking. Glass baking pans are excellent for things like casseroles and baking desserts.

- Other safer, smarter, time-tested options for pots and pans include stoneware and carbon steel cookware.

No. 2 Get Yourself a Few Helpful Kitchen Tools

Saving time in the kitchen has never been easier. When making real, fresh foods, a lot of time can be spent chopping, slicing, dicing, mincing, etc. There are incredible kitchen tools that easily do these jobs for us that are cost effective, easy to clean, and even easier to use. Some of my family's go-to kitchen tools are:

- **Multipurpose veggie chopper, dicer, etc.**
- **Peeler (great for peeling mangos, potatoes, and more)**
- **Hand frother**
- **High-speed blender**

Some of the specific kitchen tool brands we use are in the bonus resource guide as well.

No. 3 Get the Kids Involved

Just as I was heading into my office to write this chapter, I passed by my 11-year-old son, Braden, who was whipping up some eggs and a side of fresh fruit for himself. Kids have been involved in food gathering, hunting, fishing, food preparation, and cooking for countless centuries. It's only in recent decades that kids have been distanced from food preparation. And by not being involved from a young age, it's led to a decrease in people who know how to cook for themselves in young adulthood and later on in life. Data published in the *Nutrition Journal* stated: "The percentage of daily energy consumed from home food sources and time spent in food preparation decreased significantly for all socioeconomic groups between 1965 and 2008." And more recently, researchers at Tufts University found that nearly one-third of all Americans don't really know how to cook for themselves.[29,30]

The glaring <u>problem</u> is that not having this vital life skill to cook for one's self dramatically <u>increases</u> the incidence of eating fast food and ultra-<u>processed</u> prepackaged food.

The glaring problem is that not having this vital life skill to cook for one's self dramatically increases the incidence of eating fast food and ultra-processed prepackaged food, and rolling the dice every day with the food quality we are receiving. To help turn this ship around and provide our kids with this valuable gift of being able to cook and nourish their own bodies, it starts with making them feel welcome in the kitchen. In recent generations, the kitchen has become a place of isolation and territorial barriers. I, personally, had one grandmother who would allow me to see what she was doing and ask questions. And I had another grandmother who told me to get my behind out of the kitchen because it was no place for a child. Both grandmothers loved me, and both grandmothers' cooking would knock your socks off. But one of them allowed me to have *exposure* to the process of cooking, while the other only gave me the gift of her delicious cooking. That gift only carries on when we invite our kids in and allow them to help. That sometimes means things get a little more messy, take a little bit longer, or even get messed up altogether. But you get to learn and improve *together*. So get the kids involved no matter what age they're at. If they can stand on a stool next to you, they can help stir things, help measure things out, and make so many other handy kitchen contributions.

Again, invite them in, at least a couple of times a week. And most importantly, when they ask to help, find a way to say yes as often as you can. Being a parent is never about perfection, it's about progress. There have been times when my kids have asked me to help (usually when I was trying to get things done quickly) and I've said, "Not this time." But I learned to catch myself in those moments, to slow down, practice patience, and allow them to get involved more often.

No. 4   **Create the Vibe You Like**

For many families, cooking more often means doing less of something else. It's a logical trade-off that we don't usually take into account. For a new habit to stick and for a healthy, new intention to become a part of the family culture, it has to *feel* rewarding. When you try to replace something (like watching TV) with something of lesser value (like grinding away in the kitchen), then you're destined to struggle to make that healthy habit a part of your reality. As we detailed in Chapter One, a simple, psychological secret when making a habit change is to replace old habits with things that feel as though they're of equal or greater value.

If you're not passionately in love with cooking, then don't *just* cook. Intentionally add in things that *you* love while doing your thing in the kitchen. This could be blasting your favorite music and having a sing-along or dancing from ingredient to ingredient. This could be talking to a friend on the phone. This could be hanging out or cooking with someone you love. This could be popping on a weird or indulgent show that no one else will want to watch with you (my wife has been known to watch the *Real Housewives* of somewhere while cooking a time or two). There are so many possibilities to create the vibe that you enjoy. You can make it as fun, interactive, peaceful, or lively as you want to. This is practical (and powerful) and an express ticket to up-leveling your kitchen culture.

No. 5   **Store Your Food Safely**

I'm a huge fan of making enough food to have leftovers. It makes grabbing a healthy meal or snack so easy the following day or two. That said, whenever you have leftovers, storing them safely is something that more people need to know about. Plastic storage containers are the typical go-to thanks to marketing and rampant accessibility. But storing your food (especially hot food) in plastic containers is a cultural contagion that we need to move away from.

Bisphenol-A (BPA) is a noted xenoestrogen found in plastic. A xenoestrogen is a foreign estrogenic compound that's able to mimic the estrogen in our body. According to data published in *Frontiers in Bioscience*, xenoestrogens like BPA are able to bind to estrogen receptor sites in our body and disrupt the function of our endocrine system. But degeneration and leaching of the compounds in plastic are generally very minimal. So there's no need to be too neurotic when you have an occasional tryst with a plastic water bottle or container. But making plastic use a consistent practice for your food and beverages is definitely a place to have caution.[31]

A meta-analysis of over 100 studies published in the peer-reviewed journal *Environmental Research* found significant detrimental effects of BPA at even low exposures. Issues connected to BPA exposure range from infertility to obesity and more. For instance, a study published in *Fertility and Sterility* found that men with detectable levels of BPA in their system were three to four times more likely to have a low sperm concentration and low sperm count. Another study, published in *The Journal of Clinical Endocrinology and Metabolism*, found that people with the highest percentage of BPA in their system were at least 50 percent more likely to be overweight or obese. Yes, BPA-free is a step—and an acknowledgment by the plastics industry that there is a problem. But I want you to be aware that there are other concerning compounds in our conventional food and beverage packaging like bisphenol-S (BPS) and bisphenol-F (BPF). A report cited in *Environmental Health Perspectives* stated: "Based on the current literature, BPS and BPF are as hormonally active as BPA, and they have endocrine-disrupting effects."[32,33,34,35]

Just to be safe, we're going to pass on the plastics as much as possible from here on out. Here are a few awesome options for food storage that are rapidly growing in popularity:

- **Stainless-steel food storage containers**

- **Glass food storage containers**

- **Mason jars**

- **Silicone food storage containers**

One of the leading reasons people give for not cooking their own food is the cleanup afterwards. This is another area to work as a team. Just like your kids can help with cooking, they can also help with storing food and cleaning up. My wife and I do about 80 percent of the cooking and 20 percent of the cleanup/storage, while my kids do about 20 percent of the cooking and 80 percent of the cleanup/food storage. It's a formula that works for us that we figured out over time.

Remember, cooking and helping with cleanup is definitely a love language that speaks right to the heart of many people. That's why acts of service, love, and support in the kitchen can really go a long way. No matter what way your family decides to chop it up, communication, connection, and cultivating an attitude of gratitude around food and family are more important than ever right now.

Pre-Meal & Dinner Table Tips

Eating smarter and transforming family culture isn't just about what happens at the dinner table (although that's important!). It's about the daily habits we co-create together that actually build an unbreakable family foundation. Things like making healthy food choices and having healthy digestion start with the activities that occur when we're not actually eating.

Step 1 Family Fitness

Throughout our evolution, the primary driver of human movement involved the procurement of food. We moved in order to find food to eat. And we also moved in order to connect.

These genetic motivations are still alive and well within us today. We may have a society that's trying to inundate us in sedentary behavior, but tuning into what our bodies expect from us can provide a layer of resilience and health insurance for our families that's unmatched. Yes, consistent exercise is clinically proven to reduce the risk of nearly every chronic disease, radically improve our mental health, and even decrease our risk of infectious diseases. But what's left out of the conventional conversation is how much exercise influences our food choices and digestion.

A study published in the *International Journal of Obesity* found that young adults who were instructed to exercise regularly for several weeks started choosing healthier foods without being asked to. By being physically active, they automatically started making better food choices. There are many reasons why, but at its core, this is due largely to the impact that exercise has on our hormones, neurochemistry, and cognition. From a cognitive perspective, being physically active does help us to think and problem-solve better, according to data featured in the *Journal of Science & Medicine in Sport*. The researchers found that increasing access to exercise for children can improve their academic performance as well as executive mental functions like planning, cognitive flexibility, and self-control. This is a gift that we can give our kids. But there's one more benefit you need to know about.[36,37]

A recent meta-analysis published in *Oxidative Medicine and Cellular Longevity* suggests that exercise can positively enhance the number of our beneficial

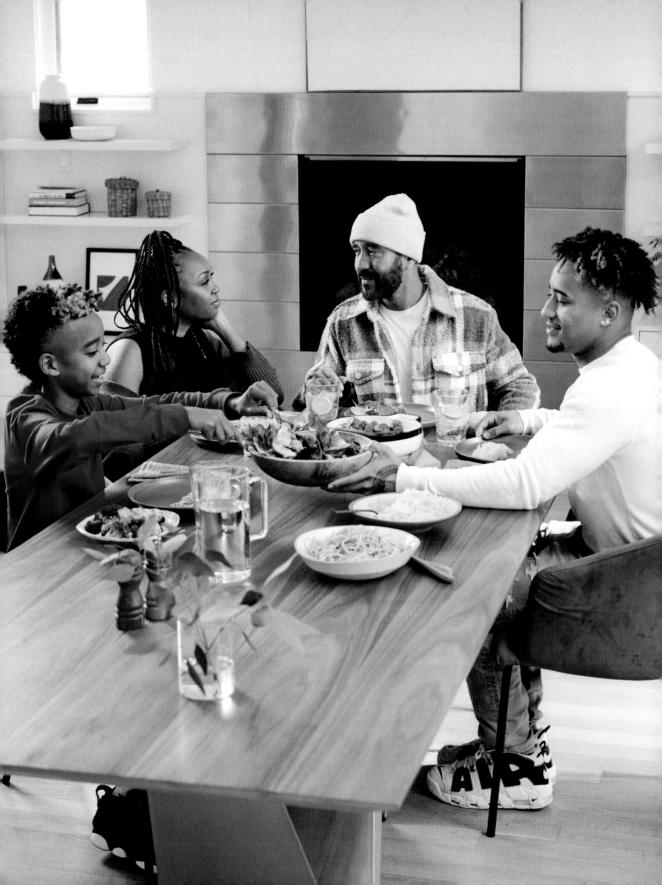

We have a chance to get exercise *off* the endangered species list and make it a part of our family culture.

microbial species, enrich our microflora diversity, and improve the development of commensal bacteria. The researchers stated: "Exercise can be used as a treatment to maintain the balance of the microflora or to rebalance [after] dysbiosis, thus obtaining an improvement of the health status." Exercise supports gut health and digestion like few things can. So many folks are investing in healthier food, but not making the most of it because they're not moving their body. Exercise radically improves the assimilation of nutrients from your food and also improves the elimination of metabolic wastes from your system.[38]

We have a chance to get exercise *off* the endangered species list and make it a part of our family culture. Several times a week, different members of my family work out together. It might be one of my sons and me, it might be my sons working out together, it might be my wife and me, or it might be a family workout with all of us. No matter what's going on with our schedule, we find ways to train together a few times a week. For years, my wife and I (together or separately) would sneak off to the gym to get a workout in. It's great that we were doing that in our own right, but my kids didn't get a chance to *witness* the workouts we were doing. And that exposure can mean everything. So when my youngest son was just a couple of years old, we started doing family workouts together at the park or track on Saturdays. It was a simple first step. We did that consistently for several years and, eventually, our culture of family fitness grew from there. It's now baked into our family recipe.

What are some ways that one or two days a week you can incorporate some family fitness into your routine? It can be anything from a family hike on Sundays, to swimming on Wednesdays after school, to moving the furniture around and exercising together with a workout video from my friend Shaun T. There are so many creative ways to build this into your family culture. Just start by selecting a special day for family fitness and make it sacred.

Step 2 **Take a Timeout from Stress**

In Chapter One, we covered some of the incredible science on how eating together with people you love can be a buffer against stress. By being more intentional about managing some of the stress in our lives, we can show up healthier and happier to the dinner table to begin with.

Ironically, when we're stressed and in need of the support of our loved ones, that stress can make us less likely to healthfully engage with them. Excessive stress can make us antisocial, irritable, and not particularly fun to be around. Plus, it can do a serious number on how food impacts our bodies. Research cited in the *Journal of Physiology and Pharmacology* details how excessive stress can lead to alterations of the gut–brain axis, ultimately leading to the development of a broad array of gastrointestinal disorders including inflammatory bowel disease, irritable bowel syndrome, food allergies, ulcers, and acid reflux. Stress can be a major culprit behind both constipation *and* diarrhea. It can back you up like a clogged faucet or it can have you evacuating like a school fire drill.[39]

Food is simply not enjoyable when your digestion is suffering. According to a report in the journal *Gastroenterology*, approximately 70 million Americans are suffering with digestive issues. This is an absolute epidemic that most folks are unaware of. And it's not just because of what we're eating, it's also because of stress.[40]

As mentioned, a major reason is because of the highly complex communication between the brain and the gut (the gut–brain axis). Researchers at the Yale University School of Medicine found that the vagus nerve communicates information between your gut and your brain about the volume and type of nutrients you have available. And depending on its perceived nutritional status, your brain can inform your gut to increase or decrease the absorption of calories and nutrients from the food you eat. This is incredibly important to understand! Based on your brain's perception of what your body has stored and what it needs, it can literally command your gut to increase or decrease the amount of calories you absorb from your food. This goes far beyond the rudimentary "calories in/calories out" paradigm to understand what actually controls what your body does with the calories you consume. There are *epicaloric controllers* ("above caloric control") that determine how your body interacts with calories to begin with.[41]

Since your brain is an epicaloric controller, what happens when there is excessive stress and dysfunction happening in your brain? Well, a recent study published in the *Annals of the New York Academy of Sciences* reported that brain inflammation is a double-edged sword to nutritional diseases. The study authors reported that systemic inflammation from things like poor metabolic health and excess body fat lead to brain inflammation, and brain inflammation, itself, leads to poor metabolic health and excess body fat. There aren't many nutrition books informing you about the importance of reducing stress and reducing brain inflammation to improve your metabolic health and reduce body fat. But this is one of the most important things you can do for your health.[42]

There are some specific foods shown to reduce brain inflammation in peer-reviewed data coming up in Chapter Three (definitely check them out!). In addition, here are some clinically proven ways to reduce your overall stress load to support your brain and digestion:

- **Meditation**
- **Walking**
- **Improving your sleep quality (there's a great book on this called *Sleep Smarter*)**
- **Music therapy**
- **Talk therapy**
- **Massage and other bodywork**
- **Engaging in healthy relationships (and eating together, of course!)**

Systemic inflammation from things like poor metabolic health and excess body fat lead to brain inflammation, and brain inflammation, itself, leads to poor metabolic health and excess body fat.

Eat Smarter

Step 3 At the Dinner Table Itself!

This is where the magic all comes together. One of the most valuable things you can do to make the most of a family meal is to take a moment to be *present*. Saying a prayer or taking a moment to give thanks is one of the underlying reasons that family meals help to center us. One of our family traditions is that, before we eat, we each share three things that we're grateful for from that day. It could be big things or small things. Anything from "I'm grateful for spending time with a friend today," "I'm grateful for getting a workout in," "I'm grateful for getting some work done on my project," to "I'm grateful for the people at the table with me." I love this family tradition because it keeps me on the lookout for things to be grateful for through the day. But you can use any family connecter you like.

Other ideas to pass around the table are:

- **Share what you're excited about**

- **Share what you're struggling with**

- **Share what you failed at today—and what you learned from it. We've done this one many times! It encourages kids to try new things, stretch themselves, and to be introspective.**

In addition to taking a moment to become present before eating, there's one more nudge for everyone to become a little more present *while* eating. A 2014 study titled "The Pathophysiology of Malabsorption" details how poor chewing has been linked to decreased nutrient absorption. And a study published in *BioMed Research International* details how the process of chewing your food well can even act as a stress reliever itself. So many wonderful meals are in our future. And we'll actually get the most from them (both the nutrition and deliciousness) by being more present, chewing well, and enjoying the process.[43,44]

Speaking of deliciousness—up next, you're about to discover some of the mind-blowing facts about the ingredients that are going to take your family's health and fitness to another level!

Eat With a Purpose

CHAPTER THREE What you eat impacts every area of your life. From your immune system to your cardiovascular system, from your metabolic health to your mental health, from the quality of your sleep to the quality of your relationships— your nutrition influences *everything about you.*

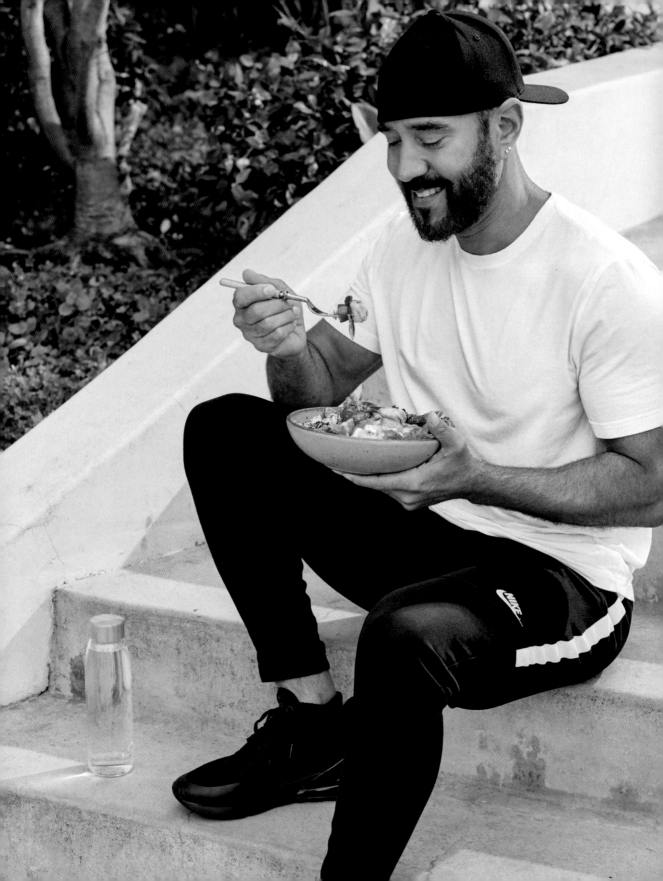

Scan here to access the bonus resource guide!

How does food affect so many things at once? We've already emphasized the fact that every single cell in your body is made from the food that you eat. But to add another layer of insight, today there are blossoming fields of *nutrigenomics* and *nutrigenetics* that are showing us how every bite of food we eat can alter our genetic expression and modify the function of every organ, tissue, and cell in our bodies. **The power isn't just in our hands; it's also at the end of our forks.**

This is the moment when you get to begin to choose your own adventure. Whatever your personal goals are—and/or the goals of your family—you can begin eating foods that fuel your specific purpose. You're about to discover the science behind specific foods and why they were intentionally used as ingredients for the recipes in the *Eat Smarter Family Cookbook*.

If your goal is to improve your memory, your focus, and boost your overall cognitive performance, you can eat foods that are clinically proven to support that. If your goal is to improve your heart health and protect your family from the leading cause of death in our world today (heart disease), you can eat amazing foods that fuel that purpose. **The benefits of each food will also be denoted by corresponding emojis:**

 = **Brain health and cognitive performance**

 = **Heart health**

 = **Metabolic health**

 = **Sleep supportive**

 = **Mental and emotional health**

 = **Gut health**

In the recipe section, you'll see these same emojis whenever their supportive ingredients are being notably utilized. This way, you'll always know what each recipe brings to the table. Keep in mind, many of these foods have wide-ranging health benefits that go beyond the power-packed science detailed here. Every food affects every cell in one way or another. We're just covering some of the biggest, brightest benefits seen in peer-reviewed research. Now let's dive into these mind-blowing food facts!

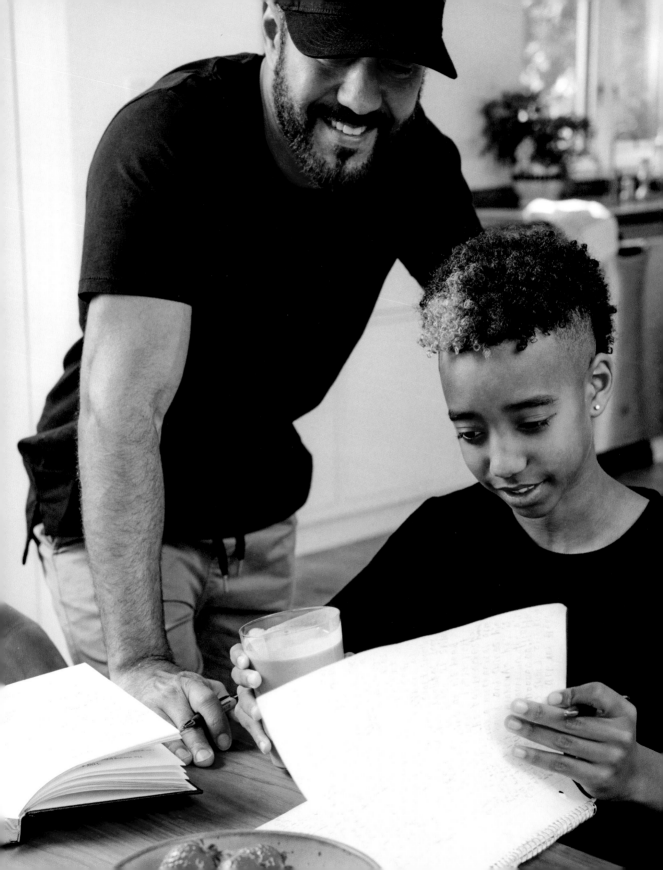

Fit Fruits

Açai

One of the most antioxidant-rich foods ever discovered, açai has remarkable potential to support our heart health and brain health, and to boost overall performance. A study published in the journal *Biology of Sport* found that açai can boost the antioxidant capacity of our blood plasma, reduce exercise-induced muscle damage, and substantially improve our ratio of blood fats. Additionally, research published in *Nutritional Neuroscience* shows that **açai has the potential to improve our memory as we age and protect our brains from excessive inflammation.**[1,2]

Blueberries

Researchers at the University of Michigan published data finding that blueberry intake can potentially affect genes related to fat burning. These little berries are a powerhouse source of micronutrients like vitamin C, vitamin K, manganese, and inflammation-fighting antioxidants. Plus, according to scientists at Harvard University the flavonoids found in blueberries were shown to be protective against weight gain. As an added bonus, it was also uncovered that having a serving of blueberries and/or strawberries three times per week can reduce your risk of having a heart attack by 34 percent. If it's good for fat loss, it's probably good for your heart, too![3,4]

If we look at the direct impact that blueberries can have on your hormones, a study published in *The Journal of Nutrition* showed that the consumption of blueberries was able to reduce insulin resistance in study participants. One more notch in blueberry's belt relates to gut health: Bifidobacteria make short-chain fatty acids that protect your gut lining and reduce inflammation. Data published in the *Journal of Agriculture and Food Chemistry* affirmed that eating blueberries increases bifidobacteria and positively modulates the diversity of gut bacteria overall.[5,6]

Cherries ♥ 💪 ☾

According to data published in the *International Journal of Food Sciences and Nutrition*, micronutrients called anthocyanins found in cherries have the potential to shrink fat cells! The researchers also noted that these **cherry anthocyanins are able to reduce the expression of genes associated with inflammation**, making them protective of your cardiovascular system. Another notable fact about cherries is their naturally occurring melatonin. A study cited in the *European Journal of Nutrition* found that tart cherries can provide exogenous melatonin that is beneficial in improving sleep duration and quality in healthy men and women. Sweet cherries have melatonin, as well, but the more tart, the more 'tonin.[7,8]

Goji Berries ♥ 💪 ⚡

A randomized, double-blind, placebo-controlled trial published in *Medicinal Chemistry* investigated the impact of goji berries on patients with type 2 diabetes. The study compared blood glucose and lipid levels of diabetic patients given goji berries compared to a diabetic control group who did not receive them. At three months into the study, it was found that patients eating goji berries had improvements in blood fat ratios with a significant increase in high-density lipoproteins (HDL) compared to controls. Moreover, their blood glucose levels decreased significantly compared to the control group as well.[9]

Several studies indicate that goji berries can also improve mental and emotional well-being. A randomized, placebo-controlled trial recently published in *Neural Regeneration Research* determined that goji berries have notable antidepressive effects.[10]

Fruits Masquerading as Vegetables

In the original bestselling book *Eat Smarter*, there is a subsection that details the little-known facts about certain fruits that are commonly thought to be vegetables in our popular culture. Fruits are often thought to be sweet, sour, and/or water rich. In reality, fruits can be fatty, savory, and even spicy! Botanically speaking, a fruit is any food that grows from a plant (vine, bush, tree, etc.) and is the means by which that plant gets its seeds out into the world. Under that definition, foods that often find themselves in the vegetable category—like zucchini, peppers, and avocados— are actually fruits. Still, from a culinary perspective, we can allow these fruits to have fake IDs to get into the veggie club if we feel inclined to. Either way, there are some phenomenal benefits found in this category that you're going to want to take advantage of!

Avocados ♥ 🦵 🌙 ⚡ ⚕

A randomized, controlled trial cited in the journal *Current Developments in Nutrition* found that **adding avocado to the diet over the course of the three-month study led to a notable reduction in abdominal fat.** Avocados are packed with sleep-supportive nutrients like potassium, vitamin B_6, and magnesium. And scientists at the University of Illinois Urbana-Champaign discovered that this wrinkly-skinned food can upgrade our diversity of gut bacteria.[11,12]

Avocados are proven to be effective in stabilizing blood sugar levels, and thereby protective of the cardiovascular system and a buffer against anxiety. Research published in the journal *Frontiers in Endocrinology* revealed that dramatic changes in blood sugar (shifting from a high blood sugar spike to an impending crash) can increase anxiety and trigger hyperactivity in the emotional centers of the brain. Studies cited in both the journals *Nutrients* and *Molecular Nutrition & Food Research* revealed that avocados can increase insulin sensitivity and improve blood sugar levels.[13,14,15]

Olives ♥ 💪 〜

Olives are one of the mightiest sources of the antioxidants oleuropein and hydroxytyrosol. They've both been shown to provide strong antioxidant and anti-inflammatory properties that reduce the risk of heart disease and defend against DNA damage. Additionally, olives deliver a variety of probiotic and prebiotic benefits.

A thirty-day clinical trial highlighted in the journal *Immunity and Aging* found that eating high-quality green olives led to reductions in oxidative stress, inflammation, and body weight for study participants. The full spectrum of olives (from green to brown to black, and everything in between) boasts similar benefits for heart health, metabolic health, and digestive wellness.[16]

Zucchini, Squash, Pumpkins, & Cucumbers 💪 〜

This camp of fruits in vegetable clothing provides a vast array of micronutrients and prebiotic fiber types that support satiety and overall metabolic health. One of the most studied satiety-related hormones, adiponectin, has been shown to support fat loss while simultaneously keeping appetite in check. A meta-analysis of 52 studies uncovered that by simply increasing fiber intake you can boost adiponectin levels by 60 to 115 percent![17]

Zucchini, squash, pumpkins, cucumbers, and other members of the gourd family have been shown to be supportive of microbiome diversity and blood sugar regulation. For instance, a study published in the peer-reviewed journal *BioImpacts* found that cucumbers may be effective at reducing oxidative stress and preventing complications related to diabetes.[18]

Vital Veggies

Asparagus ♥ 💪 ≋

These green spears are a generally common food that feature a great amount of the prebiotic fiber inulin. In a fascinating study published in the journal *Gut*, inulin-derived propionate was found to significantly increase the release of PYY (peptide YY) and GLP-1 (glucagon-like peptide-1), two of our body's major hormones regulating satiety and metabolism. Eating prebiotic plant fibers from foods like asparagus has been found to produce substantial gut protection and anti-inflammatory properties. Several studies indicate nutrients in asparagus have free radical scavenging abilities that can reduce the risk of heart disease.[19]

Broccoli 🧠 💪

This cruciferous veggie is an excellent source of nutrients called isothiocyanates. These remarkable compounds have been found to help reduce brain inflammation and provide protection against neurodegenerative diseases. As far as metabolic health is concerned, a process called aromatization can "rob" androgenic hormones and convert them into more estrogen in both men and women. Data published in the peer-reviewed journal *Anti-Cancer Agents in Medicinal Chemistry* found that compounds in cruciferous vegetables like broccoli are able to effectively block excess aromatization from taking place. You may be curious why this information is cited in a journal that's dedicated to cancer research, and the answer is because this category of foods is also a potent defense against estrogen-driven cancers.[20,21]

Brussels Sprouts ♥ 💪 ☾

As a standout member of the cruciferous family, eating Brussels sprouts may significantly reduce the risk of developing type 2 diabetes, according to a study published in the journal *Primary Care Diabetes*. Brussels sprouts are rich in a variety of antioxidants that help neutralize free radicals, reduce inflammation, and help protect cardiovascular health. They're also exceptionally high in the immune-

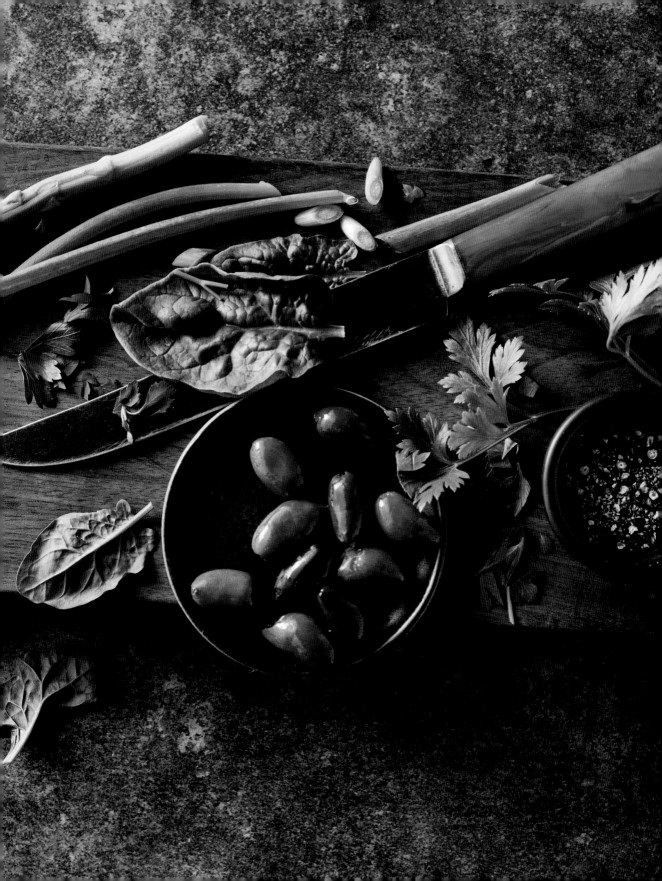

supportive, good-sleep nutrient vitamin C. Data cited in the journals *Appetite* and *PLoS One* demonstrated that insufficient intake of vitamin C increases the likelihood of sleep disturbances and shortens the duration of overall sleep time. This low-glycemic little veggie is a great way to boost vitamin C while keeping blood sugar levels in check.[22,23,24]

Kimchi 💪🐍

Heavily studied the last few years for its remarkable antiobesity benefits, kimchi is gaining massive popularity outside of its original home in Korea. Kimchi is a spicy, fermented vegetable side dish that has a base of cabbage and can include an assortment of other ingredients like ginger, garlic, daikon radishes, carrots, red pepper, fish sauce, scallions, and more.

A peer-reviewed study published in the journal *Nutrition Research* found that **eating kimchi led to a significant decrease in body fat, hip-to-waist ratio, and fasting blood sugar for study participants** versus those who merely ate the unfermented form of the cabbage dish. Something really cool happens when the bacteria integrate with it, and it has positive effects on our metabolism. One of the reasons that I really love kimchi is that it's a great source of friendly flora that also comes along with the prebiotic fiber from the vegetables. Having three to four servings of fermented veggies like kimchi each week is supportive of both your gut health and your metabolism.[25]

Spinach 🧠💪

A study published in the journal *Appetite* uncovered that compounds found in green leafy vegetables like spinach were able to significantly increase post-meal levels of the satiety hormone GLP-1 in study participants. This corresponded with a greater reduction in weight, body fat, and waist circumference over the course of the twelve-week study period.

Scientists at Chicago's Rush University Medical Center found that people who ate one to two servings of leafy green vegetables like spinach each day experienced fewer memory problems and less cognitive decline. Compared to people who rarely ate leafy greens, study participants who ate about two servings a day had brains that were roughly eleven years younger![26,27]

Sea Veggies 💜 💪 ☾

Our oceans are home to some of the last truly wild foods that humans regularly consume. Many cultures have prized the benefits of seaweeds (lovingly referred to as sea veggies) for centuries, and for good reason. One of the most fascinating micronutrients found in sea veggies like wakame, hijiki, and kelp is a compound called fucoxanthin. Research cited in the journal *Food Science and Human Wellness* asserts that **seaweeds have antiobesity effects that can improve metabolic rate and increase satiety.** Specifically, the seaweed carotenoid, fucoxanthin was found to boost the activity of uncoupling protein 1 (UCP1) that enhances the activity of brown adipose tissue (a type of fat that *burns* excess fat), while simultaneously supporting the reduction of belly fat from the waistline.[28]

According to the US Department of Agriculture, kelp has more calcium than just about all other vegetables, and gram for gram, kelp contains even more calcium than milk. Research published in the *International Journal of Obesity* determined that adequate calcium intake can downregulate enzymes that create fat *and* potentially decrease levels of blood fats. Other sea veggies include dulse, arame, sea lettuce, and nori, among many others. Rich in selenium and zinc, plus good-sleep nutrients like potassium, magnesium, and B vitamins, sea veggies might just be the most micronutrient-dense foods on the planet.[29]

Sweet Potatoes 🧠 💪 ⚕

Several studies have found that the soluble fiber in sweet potatoes can provide excellent support for overall gut health. The prebiotic fibers support the production of short-chain fatty acids that protect the gut lining and reduce systemic inflammation. As for metabolic benefits, a recent study published in the journal *Nutrients* specifically analyzed the inclusion of sweet potatoes on a macro-managed, calorie-restricted diet. The participants who included sweet potato as part of their diet lost more weight and body fat than the control group. Plus, the sweet potato group had a greater drop in glycated hemoglobin levels (HbA1c), a marker for risk of insulin resistance and diabetes.[30,31,32]

Not to be left out, having a potato head might actually be a good thing. An analysis published in *Archives of Pharmacal Research* revealed that anthocyanins in sweet potato exhibit memory-enhancing effects. The researchers believe this is due to its potent antioxidant effects.[33]

Powerful Proteins

Eggs 🧠 💪

Studies published in both the *International Journal of Obesity* and the journal *Nutrients* determined that *eating eggs for the first meal of the day can improve levels of satiety hormones, reduce levels of the hunger-hormone ghrelin, and enhance overall weight loss.*[34,35]

Choline is one of the most important things for developing your lifelong memory capabilities. Research conducted by scientists at the University of North Carolina postulates that your memory characteristics are heavily impacted by how much choline your mother ate during pregnancy and lactation. Choline is still important to the memory center of your brain throughout life, and one of the very best places to find it is egg yolks. Now, egg yolks have gone in and out of fashion more times than short shorts and fanny packs. But the myths around eggs and heart disease have been put to bed yet again by researchers from the Department of Nutritional Sciences at the University of Connecticut. Their data concluded that eating whole eggs, specifically, does not translate to increased risk of heart disease and problematic ratios of cholesterol. In fact, eating eggs was found to *decrease* heart disease risk.[36,37]

Free-Range Chicken 🧠 💪

Unlike newly invented ultra-processed foods, humans have included chicken in our diet for at least 10,000 years. One of the regions noted to make chicken a staple thousands of years ago is the Mediterranean. The coveted Mediterranean diet is far more diverse than people realize. Yet from country to country and town to town, you'll likely find chicken as part of the cuisine. Italian scientists, in a meta-analysis published in the journal *Food & Nutrition Research*, determined that the inclusion of chicken as part of a balanced, whole food–based diet is associated with a significant reduction in the risk of developing obesity, type 2 diabetes, and cardiovascular diseases. The researchers also noted the abundance of bioavailable amino acids and micronutrients found in chicken. These key nutrients have been found to improve cognitive function, boost the activity of satiety hormones, and support the growth and maintenance of muscle tissue.[38]

Grass-Fed Beef

A 16-week study published in the journal *Obesity Science & Practice* found that increasing the ratio of dietary protein–with one group *specifically* including more beef–led to substantial weight loss *and* fat loss for overweight and obese participants. Not only did the test subjects see an improvement in their cardiometabolic health, they also maintained their existing muscle mass, which is frequently reduced with conventional weight loss diets.[39]

According to a study cited in the *European Journal of Clinical Nutrition*, improving zinc levels may be effective in reducing anger and depression. Beef is loaded with zinc that keeps brain nerves calm, reining in worry, chronic tension, and stress, explained study coauthor Dr. Takako Sawada. Not only that—beef is at the top of the list for the amino acid glycine. A study reported in *Neuropsychopharmacology* revealed that glycine appears to improve deep sleep time and reduce waking after sleep onset (meaning you wake up less often).[40,41]

Grass-Fed Whole Milk Yogurt

An expansive analysis published in the *British Journal of Nutrition* revealed that fermented dairy products like yogurt have a protective effect against glucose impairment seen in diabetes and prediabetes. Moreover, a multiyear study that included over 18,000 women found that a greater intake of specifically *high-fat* dairy products, including yogurt, was associated with less weight gain than in study participants consuming low-fat dairy products.[42,43]

Yogurt has been prized for centuries for its benefits to digestive health. Recently, scientists at the University of Maryland School of Medicine discovered that yogurt has protective effects when the microbiome is exposed to antibiotic use. Finally, yogurt is an excellent source of good-sleep nutrients like vitamin B_6. Vitamin B_6 is a crucial cofactor in the tryptophan–serotonin pathway. This essential vitamin helps to modulate our body's stress response, relax the nervous system, and even helps improve sleep quality.[44]

Mahi Mahi & Other Lean Fish

A lot of the health conversation revolves around fatty fish like salmon—and for good reason as you'll learn more about shortly. But the truth is, lean fish like mahi mahi, halibut, and cod provide some remarkable benefits as well. A study published in the *Journal of Nutrition* found that the inclusion of white fish helps optimize satiety hormones and can be significantly more satiating than other dense protein foods. Another study published in the *International Journal of Obesity* put test subjects on a reduced-calorie diet that included either cod, salmon, or no fish. Even though the macronutrient content of all the diets was the same, simply including **three 5-ounce servings of fish per week resulted in study participants losing over 2 additional pounds within four weeks.** Again, same amount of calories, same macronutrient ratio, but including fish did something extra for their metabolism.[45,46]

Lean fish is rich in amino acids and micronutrients like selenium and B_{12} that are essential for energy production, cognitive performance, and mental health. Taking a look at the impact of B_{12}, for example, an analysis published in *The American Journal of Psychiatry* determined that a B_{12} deficiency could potentially *double* the risk of severe depression. Lean fish can truly be a bona fide brain friend with benefits.[47]

Spirulina

Spirulina has been a major protein source for human civilizations spanning thousands of years. Its use has been traced back to the ancient Aztecs of Mesoamerica, but more recently its potential has jumped light-years ahead with NASA initiating research proposing this nutrient-dense algae could be utilized by astronauts in space.[48]

Spirulina is approximately 71 percent protein by weight, and proven to be beneficial for both the brain and metabolic health. A recent study published in *PLoS One* revealed that **spirulina has the potential to improve neurogenesis in the brain** *and* **reduce neuroinflammation.** A separate double-blind, placebo-controlled study found that participants who utilized spirulina lost more weight and had a greater reduction in BMI than those taking a placebo.[49,50]

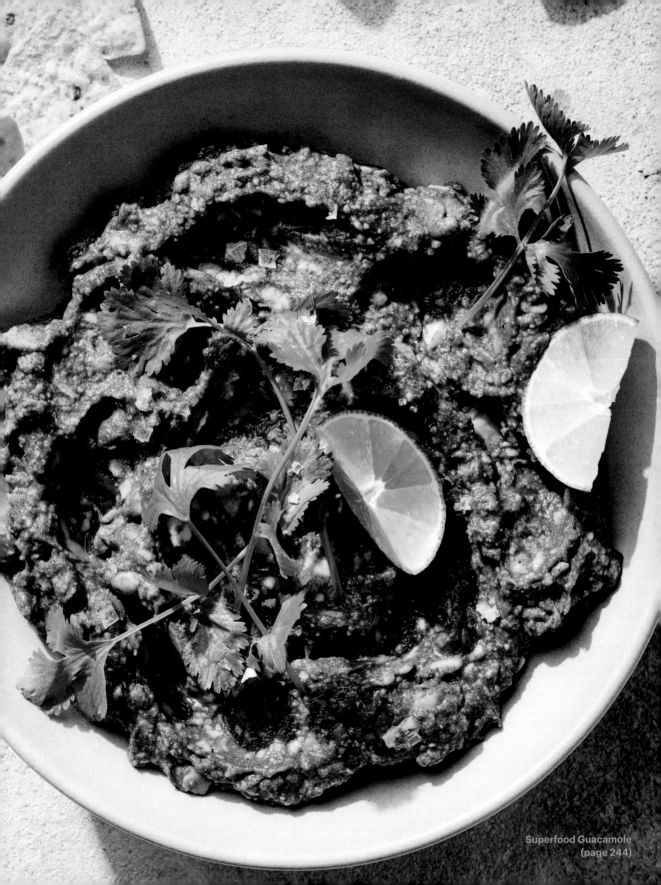

Superfood Guacamole
(page 244)

Whey Protein 🧠 💪 ⚡

Whey protein may seem relatively new, but it has origins dating back thousands of years. Even Hippocrates, who's widely considered to be the father of modern medicine, prized whey as a treatment for his patients to restore vitality and boost the immune system.

A randomized double-blind study published in the *Journal of Nutrition* observed that overweight participants who were instructed to consume whey protein daily for twenty-three weeks lost more fat mass, had a greater loss in waist circumference, and had a greater reduction of circulating ghrelin levels (the major hunger hormone) compared to test subjects taking daily soy protein or an isogenic carbohydrate drink. What's really interesting about this study is that the test subjects were not instructed to make any other dietary or lifestyle changes. Just adding in more protein led to these results. Again, more satiety from our nutrition leads to less likelihood of hanger (hungry + anger/irritation) showing up. Even in individuals who are more vulnerable to stress, research published in the *American Journal of Clinical Nutrition* found that whey protein consumption improved their coping ability and boosted their overall cognitive performance.[51,52]

Wild-Caught Salmon 🧠 ❤️ 💪 🌙 ⚡

Thanks in large part to its concentration of protein, an eight-week randomized controlled trial published in the journal *Nutrition* revealed that the inclusion of salmon multiple times each week led to significant reductions in blood pressure and body weight for overweight individuals.[53]

Fatty fish are a rich source of docosahexaenoic acid (DHA) and eicosapentaenoic acid (EPA), omega-3 fats that are critical for maintenance of the brain and nervous system. This is why fish like salmon can improve cognition and mental well-being. Researchers at Rush University Medical Center uncovered that adults who eat at least one seafood meal per week do, in fact, perform better on cognitive skills tests than people who consume less. Additionally, a meta-analysis published in *Translational Psychiatry* found that the omega-3s in fatty fish (specifically EPA) have a beneficial overall effect on individuals with major depressive disorders.[54,55]

Health Nuts (and Seeds)

Almonds ♥ 💪 ☾

A study cited in the *Journal of Research in Medical Sciences* put participants on matching reduced-calorie diets for three months, with one interesting difference: one group included almonds in their diet, while the other group did not. After the data was compiled at the end of the study, the folks who included almonds in their diet lost *twice* as much weight and had a greater reduction in their hip-to-waist ratio than those in the almond-free group! The researchers found a greater improvement in insulin sensitivity and satiety hormones in the almond group.[56]

Almonds are also heart healthy. Data published in *The Journal of Nutrition* found that eating almonds decreases the risk of oxidative damage. To top things off, almonds are a great source of sleep-supportive micronutrients like magnesium, calcium, B vitamins, and vitamin E.[57]

Chia Seeds ♥ ☾ ⚡ ⚖

Multiple studies indicate that chia seeds can be helpful in regulating blood sugar and improving metabolic health. To that point, **a double-blind randomized controlled trial published in 2017 found that participants who included chia seeds in their diet lost more weight and more belly fat than the control group.** The study also noted a greater decrease in C-reactive protein, indicating reduced inflammation and reduced risk of cardiovascular disease.[58]

A fascinating study published in the journal *Nutrients* uncovered that chia seeds can potentially improve intestinal health and functionality and improve the absorption of essential minerals. And speaking of essential minerals, chia seeds are a top-notch source of calcium and magnesium, both noted for the ability to improve sleep quality.[59]

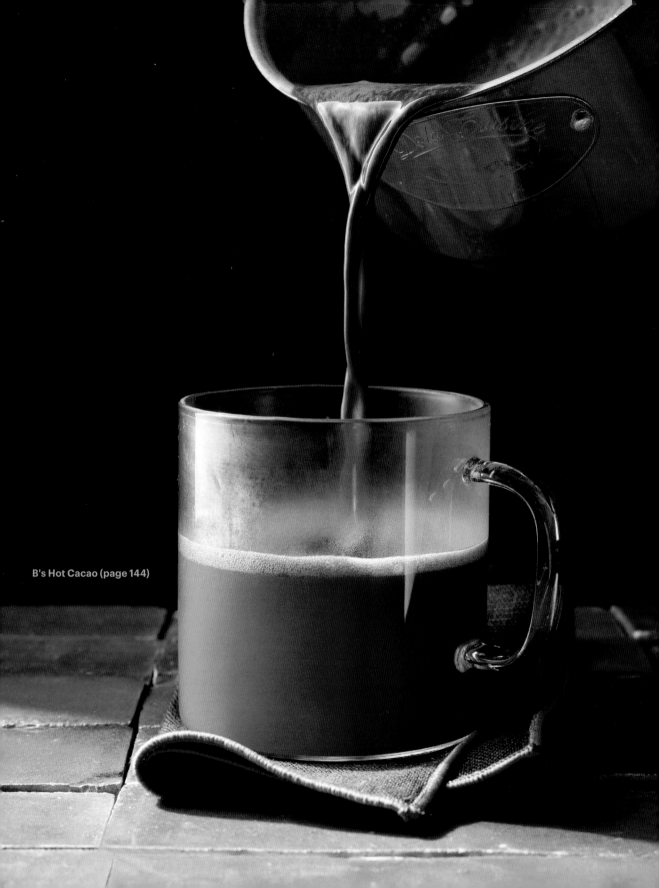

B's Hot Cacao (page 144)

Chocolate ⦿ ♥ ☾ ⚡ ≋

The world's most popular seed (although most folks don't realize it's a seed) is packed with some serious nutrition that's detailed in hundreds of peer-reviewed studies. Similar to apple seeds or pumpkin seeds, cacao "beans" (the basis of all chocolate) are the seeds of a fruit as well–known as cacao fruit. Depending upon how the cacao beans are used, they can be shaped into nutrient-dense superfoods or ultra-processed junk foods. The choice is up to us.

A randomized double-blind controlled study published by the *American Journal of Clinical Nutrition* revealed that polyphenol-rich cacao powder has remarkable prebiotic effects in the human body. Study participants consuming a sugar-free cacao flavanol drink for four weeks significantly increased their ratio of bifidobacteria and lactobacilli populations, while significantly *decreasing* their counts of clostridia (a class of bacteria associated with fat gain). These microbial changes were paralleled by significant reductions in plasma triglycerides (blood fats) and C-reactive protein concentrations, indicating reduced inflammation and cardiovascular protection.[60]

Another study conducted by researchers at Columbia University Irving Medical Center found that chocolate has strong potential to protect your brain against age-related memory loss, while a study published in the *International Journal of Health Sciences* determined that a small amount of chocolate can significantly decrease perceived stress. And, to top it off, chocolate is one of the richest sources of magnesium and tryptophan, two outstanding good-sleep nutrients.[61,62]

Hemp Seeds ♥ ≋

One of the special things about hemp seeds is that they're one of the rare complete protein sources you'll find within a single plant. Hemp seeds are upwards of 25 to 30 percent protein by weight, and have an excellent ratio of essential fatty acids, as well. The primary omega-3 you'll find in hemp seeds and other plant sources is alpha-linolenic acid (ALA), which is noted for being protective of your heart and nervous system. But hemp seeds also contain gamma-linolenic acid (GLA), which, according to data cited in the journal *Inflammation*, has significant anti-inflammatory properties.[63]

Promising research from the *American Journal of Physiology* also shows potential in hemp seeds to support recovery after cardiovascular injuries. In addition, a growing body of data shows that hemp seeds may have significant benefits for our microbiome.[64]

Pumpkin Seeds ♥ 💪 🌙 ⚡

These tasty seeds are a great source of several good sleep nutrients like magnesium, omega-3s, and tryptophan. Improving tryptophan levels has been shown to reduce wakefulness at night, improve the quality of REM sleep, and increase mental alertness after waking up in the morning, according to research cited in the journal *Nutrients*. It's also important to note that tryptophan is a precursor for making your body's feel-good neurotransmitter serotonin. And serotonin is a precursor for making the sleep-regulating superstar melatonin.[65]

Several studies have revealed that compounds in pumpkin seeds have benefits for heart health. And a study cited in the peer-reviewed publication *Journal of Diabetes and Its Complications* found that pumpkin seeds have the potential to help reduce blood glucose levels and provide other antiobesity effects as well.[66]

Quinoa ♥ 💪 🌙

Quinoa has been prized as a food for thousands of years. Technically, quinoa is the seed of the Chenopodium quinoa plant, but because of its similar nutrient profile to grains and the way that it's used culinarily, it's often classified as a grain. You can refer to quinoa as a seed, grain, or pseudograin. Just make sure to put some respect on its nutrient profile.;)

Researchers from the Department of Food Science and Microbiology at the University of Milan uncovered that quinoa reduced blood sugar and triglyceride levels more than any grain it was tested against. And according to data published in the journal *Plant Foods for Human Nutrition*, quinoa appears to have cardiometabolic benefits that even reduce the impact that highly refined sweeteners have on our bodies. It's important to note that quinoa is another one of the very few plant-based foods that are also complete proteins. Plus, it's rich in micronutrients like magnesium and vitamin B_6, two of the most valuable good-sleep nutrients.[67,68]

Walnuts 🧠 ♥ 🦴

Compounds found in walnuts have been shown to help scrub your brain clear of the harmful amyloid beta peptide that leads to certified amyloid plaque build-up. The data, highlighted in the journal *Neurochemical Research*, demonstrated that walnuts have the potential to reduce oxidative stress, reduce inflammation, and protect your brain cells from an early demise. What's more, recent research from UCLA suggests that **eating a handful of walnuts per day may help boost memory, concentration, and the speed at which your brain processes information.**[69,70]

Walnuts are the king of the omega-3 ALA in the nut family. Research published in the *American Journal of Clinical Nutrition* states that each gram of ALA you eat per day lowers your risk of dying from heart disease by 10 percent. And to add a finishing touch to this nutty superstar, the polyphenols in walnuts make them fantastically heart healthy and gut healthy. A randomized controlled cross-over study found that eating walnuts significantly improves microbiome composition and diversity.[71,72]

Fantastic Fats

Coconut Oil

A study published in the journal *Experimental and Therapeutic Medicine* describes coconut oil as an "antistress functional oil." The researchers found that antioxidants and antioxidant-potentiators in coconut oil have the potential to protect our brains under stress and even exhibit antidepressant qualities.[73]

The fats in coconut oil are incredibly stable and less prone to oxidation or rancidity than lesser saturated fats. Coconut oil is approximately 65 percent medium chain triglycerides (MCTs, which you'll learn more about in a moment) that provide notable brain and metabolism-supportive benefits.

Grass-Fed Butter

Butter is another food eaten by humans for thousands of years that fell out of favor due to the haphazard war on dietary fats. What make butter so advantageous is its diversity of fats, its limited number of potential allergens (since the milk sugars and proteins are removed), and its stability at different temperatures. One of the extraordinary things about butter is its rich concentration of conjugated linoleic acid (CLA) and its influence on metabolism.

In a surprising meta-analysis that included more than 630,000 study participants, published in the peer-reviewed journal *PLoS One*, it was found that for each tablespoon of butter included in their daily diet they saw an additional 4 percent reduction in their risk for type 2 diabetes. A new randomized double-blind study found that the CLA in butter is able to reduce levels of several proteins involved in inflammation, including tumor necrosis factor and C-reactive protein. If you'd like to include butter in your personal nutrition protocol, it's important to keep the data in mind from the scientists at the University of Wisconsin–Madison indicating that grass-fed butter contains up to 500 percent more CLA than conventional grain-fed butter.[74,75,76]

MCT Oil

Medium chain triglycerides (MCTs) are getting a lot of attention right now for their wide-ranging benefits on brain health and metabolism. A randomized double-blind study published in the *International Journal of Obesity and Related Metabolic Disorders* placed participants on a reduced-calorie diet that included either supplemental MCTs or supplemental long chain triglycerides (LCTs). After the data was compiled, it was revealed that the group who included MCT oil lost more weight, eliminated more body fat, and experienced higher levels of satiety. What was particularly interesting about this study was that people consuming MCTs were able to retain more of their muscle mass during the weight-loss process.[77]

Researchers at Yale University published data affirming that MCTs can readily cross the blood-brain barrier and be utilized by brain cells. Another study, featured in the *Annals of the New York Academy of Sciences*, found that the consumption of MCTs directly led to improved cognitive function in patients with mild to moderate forms of Alzheimer's disease and cognitive impairment.[78,79]

Olive Oil

Groundbreaking research published in *ACS Chemical Neuroscience* asserts that *extra virgin olive oil has the ability to reduce brain inflammation, improve autophagy (self-cleaning/regeneration) in the brain, and improve the function of the blood-brain barrier.* Well noted for its cardiovascular benefits, numerous studies also show that olive oil supports healthy cholesterol ratios and reduces rates of hypertension.[80]

Another recent study cited in the *American Journal of Clinical Nutrition* revealed that consuming a little more than a tablespoon of olive oil triggered the release of not one but *three* of the major satiety hormones associated with enhanced fat loss. A separate double-blind placebo-controlled trial had overweight test subjects consume a breakfast that contained about 1½ tablespoons extra virgin olive oil or 1½ tablespoons soybean oil as part of an overall reduced-calorie diet. At the end of the study, they found that test subjects given the extra virgin olive oil lost 80 percent more body fat![81,82]

Beverages

Charged Water 🧠 💜 🦵 🌙 ⚡ 🦴

It's so simple, yet so overlooked. Optimal hydration impacts every single area of our health more powerfully than almost anything else. Take its impact on our brain and cognitive performance. Most people don't realize that **insufficient hydration is the number one nutritive trigger of daytime fatigue.** Recent data published in the *International Journal of Environmental Research and Public Health* revealed that mild dehydration had a significant negative impact on fatigue, mood, reading speed, and mental work capacity in collegiate test subjects. Within a short amount of time, getting them properly hydrated alleviated fatigue, improved total mood disturbance, boosted short-term memory, and enhanced their focus and reaction times.[83]

It's critical to understand that **none of the processes of metabolism can take place without the presence of water.** It is truly that important. Simply drinking water provides an immediate boost to your metabolism because it makes everything work better. A simple illustration of this is noted in a study published in the *Journal of Clinical Endocrinology and Metabolism* finding that drinking water can increase your metabolic rate through a process called water-induced thermogenesis. From your neurons, to hormones, to your mitochondria (where fat is actually burned), they're all operating in a water medium. Without proper hydration (along with electrolytes that provide an electric "charge"), all of these systems become stagnant and inefficient.[84]

Coffee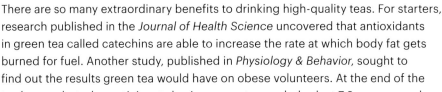

A recent study featured in the journal *Practical Neurology* details how regularly drinking coffee has been shown to help prevent cognitive decline and reduce the risk of developing Alzheimer's and Parkinson's diseases. In a sip beyond that, scientists at Stanford University recently deduced that the caffeine in coffee is able to defend against age-related inflammation. Their research revealed that light to moderate coffee drinkers live longer and more healthfully, thanks in part to the protection caffeine provides by suppressing genes related to inflammation.[85,86]

When quality is honored, there are some absolutely mind-blowing benefits to drinking coffee. And skipping the pesticides and high glycemic sweeteners found in the typical cup of joe can actually help stack conditions in your metabolic favor. After adjusting for a variety of lifestyle factors, a study published in the journal *Nutrition* found that light to moderate coffee drinkers (one to four cups per day) had the lowest amounts of visceral belly fat compared to non-coffee drinkers and heavy coffee drinkers. Plus, scientists from the School of Medicine at the University of Nottingham discovered that coffee may be able to influence the activity of your brown adipose tissue (the type of fat that *burns* excess fat). The researchers used thermal imaging and found that drinking coffee lights up brown fat–dominant locations on the body, indicating increased thermogenesis.[87,88]

Black, Green & Herbal Teas

There are so many extraordinary benefits to drinking high-quality teas. For starters, research published in the *Journal of Health Science* uncovered that antioxidants in green tea called catechins are able to increase the rate at which body fat gets burned for fuel. Another study, published in *Physiology & Behavior,* sought to find out the results green tea would have on obese volunteers. At the end of the twelve-week study, participants having green tea each day lost 7.3 more pounds and burned 183 more calories per day than those who didn't have green tea, even though they were eating the same calorie-controlled meals![89,90]

A group of polyphenols found in higher concentration in black tea called theaflavins appear to have some remarkable benefits on metabolism as well. Research cited in the *Journal of Functional Foods* revealed that black tea theaflavins have the ability to literally shift human gene expression to a profile that favors lipolysis and beta oxidation (burning fat for fuel!). To highlight this, scientists at the University of Oslo in Norway conducted a double-blind placebo-controlled study and found that the **participants drinking black tea lost significantly more weight**

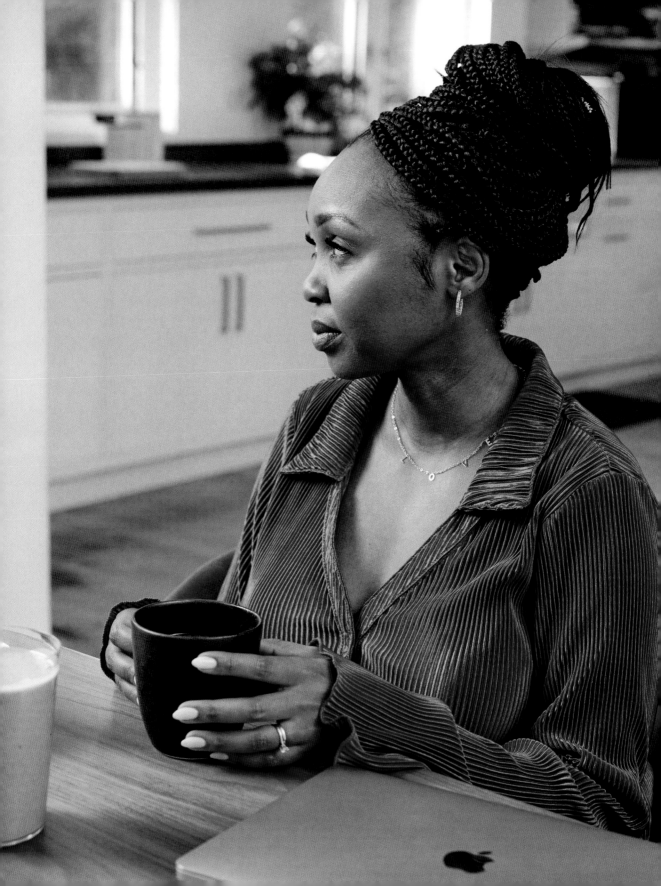

and had a greater reduction in waist circumference after the three-month study period. Both black and green tea are well noted to significantly reduce your risk of cardiovascular disease.[91,92]

There are so many remarkable herbal teas as well. One of my favorites is rooibos (pronounced ROY-boss). Boasting upwards of 50 percent more antioxidants than even green tea, this caffeine-free tea has been found to improve insulin sensitivity and even block the creation of new fat cells, as detailed in a recent study published in *Phytomedicine*. All of these teas are well noted to support our mental well-being and cognitive performance. Rooibos is shown to reduce anxiety and provide neuroprotection against stress, while green and black tea are some of the richest sources of L-theanine. In a study published in the journal *Brain Topography*, researchers observed that L-theanine intake increases the frequency of alpha brain waves, indicating reduced stress, enhanced focus, and even increased creativity.[93,94]

Spices of Life

Cinnamon

Scientists at UC Santa Barbara discovered that phytonutrients in cinnamon can help lower the risk of Alzheimer's disease by reducing tangles of tau proteins in the brain. Their data showed that cinnamon can inhibit these tangles from happening in the first place, lower oxidative stress, and improve the overall health of neurons. Another study cited in the *Journal of Neuroimmune Pharmacology* discovered that cinnamon has the potential to improve the learning speed of folks with learning challenges by stimulating hippocampal plasticity.[95,96]

A meta-analysis of randomized controlled trials published in the journal *Diabetes, Obesity & Metabolism* revealed some remarkable effects that cinnamon can have on blood sugar. The analysis showed that cinnamon can potentially lower fasting blood sugar levels by 18 to 29 percent in folks with insulin resistance. Keep in mind, special foods and spices that help stabilize your blood sugar can also stabilize your mood. **Researchers at The Ohio State University found that abnormal blood sugar levels caused couples to feel angrier and more aggressive towards their partners.** Not only can cinnamon improve insulin sensitivity, but it can also decrease the amount of glucose that enters your bloodstream after a meal as well.[97,98]

Garlic

A myriad of randomized placebo-controlled trials have found that garlic can improve cardiovascular health by improving endothelial function, boosting antioxidant status, and reducing oxidative stress. In addition, research cited in the journal *Food Science and Human Wellness* noted garlic's potential as a prebiotic and protection against digestive diseases. And one more little bulb of benefit featured in the journal *Drug and Chemical Toxicology* revealed that garlic can help improve memory and learning speed, even when brain cells are damaged from toxin exposure.[99,100,101]

Onions

One of the most decorated spices in the world, onions are also one of the most revered prebiotic foods that support your friendly gut flora. Onions have been found to aid gut bacteria in making the short chain fatty acid propionate. Not only is propionate noted for its ability to reduce inflammation, but it can also be helpful in reducing visceral belly fat![102,103]

Antioxidants like quercetin found in onions provide phenomenal benefits for our heart health. A randomized placebo-controlled trial found that an onion extract was able to significantly reduce the blood pressure of participants with hypertension over the course of a six-week study period.[104]

Honey

It's impossible to classify honey as merely a spice or sweetener. There really is nothing else like it on Earth. Unlike other sweeteners, raw honey has been found to actually *improve* insulin sensitivity. A recent study published in the peer-reviewed journal *Nutrients* detailed how raw honey intake can improve fasting blood sugar levels, improve lipid metabolism, and reduce the risk of heart disease. Additionally, the scientists noted the vast antioxidant and anti-inflammatory properties that honey has.[105]

Research cited in the journal *Evidence-Based Complementary and Alternative Medicine* determined that honey antioxidants have nootropic effects such as memory enhancement. Plus, a randomized double-blind placebo-controlled study revealed that honey was able to outperform a placebo and significantly reduce cough frequency and severity and improve sleep quality.[106,107]

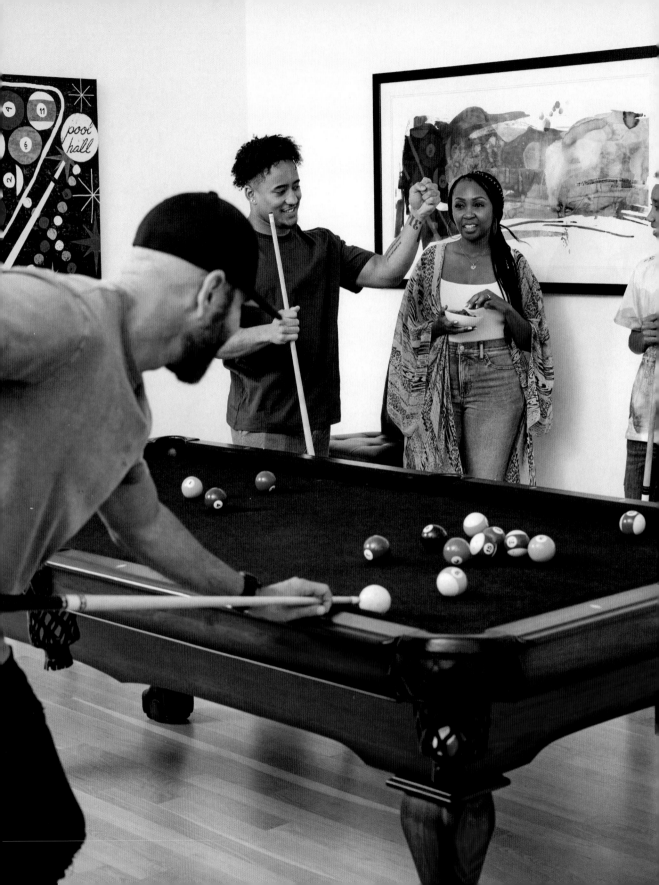

Salt 🧠 💪

A study conducted by researchers at Harvard Medical School and published in the journal *Metabolism* found that low salt intake directly increases insulin resistance in healthy test subjects. Salt is shown to support cellular communication and improve the function of many of our major hormones. Additionally, research cited in *Scientific Reports* revealed that a low-salt diet could increase levels of the hunger hormone ghrelin.[108,109]

Salt provides one of the most important electrolytes for brain health and cognitive function. Standard salt is 40 percent sodium. Not only is sodium critical to maintaining proper fluid balance in the brain, a study conducted by researchers at McGill University found that sodium functions as an "on/off switch" in the brain for specific neurotransmitters that support optimal function and protect the brain against numerous diseases.[110]

Turmeric 🧠 💗 💪 ⚡

Scientists from the Department of Neurology at USC found that curcumin, one of the active ingredients in turmeric, is able to help eliminate amyloid plaque, slow down the aging of neurons, excavate heavy metals, and reduce inflammation in the brain. Another study, published in the *European Journal of Nutrition*, uncovered that compounds in turmeric can downregulate inflammatory cytokines and upregulate the activity of adiponectin and other satiety-related hormones.[111,112]

Turmeric has also been found to improve insulin sensitivity, reduce blood fats, and directly act upon fat cells. Plus, research published in the *Journal of Ethnopharmacology* points to turmeric's potential in reducing severity of both anxiety and depression.[113]

There are many other powerful, purposeful ingredients included in the recipes (some of the recipe descriptions will make note of them). But the food facts we just covered are to further spark the power and influence you have in determining your destiny through the foods you choose. Understanding *why* we're using the foods that we're using is a huge key to internal motivation, consistent application, and transformative results!

Start the Day with Momentum!

I love the Aristotelian quote that says, "We are what we repeatedly do. Excellence, therefore, is not an act, but a habit." When it comes to creating a healthy culture, it's not what you do every now and then, it's what you do on a consistent basis. How we start our days sets the tone for how the day will unfold. If we can implement a few smarter daily habits, we can create a health-affirming momentum that's unstoppable.

No. 1 Take an Inner Bath

While we are asleep, our bodies undertake hundreds of different processes to repair damaged tissues, fortify our immune system, eliminate old cells, and more. All of this results in a tremendous amount of metabolic waste products that need to be removed. Drinking water when you wake up literally helps to flush these things out, or you'll risk them slowing your metabolism down like a hormonal clog. And just logically speaking, your hydration levels are lower due to the sheer amount of time you've gone without water while you're asleep for several hours. When you wake up, your body needs water first. Not coffee. Not SunnyD. Water.

Plus, you'll also receive that metabolic boost via water-induced thermogenesis that we talked about earlier in Chapter Three. The study we noted, published in the *Journal of Clinical Endocrinology and Metabolism*, revealed that by drinking about 17 ounces of water within a couple of minutes of rising you can temporarily boost your metabolic rate by about 30 percent! This helps to put your metabolic systems in the ON position to start the day. It's a huge advantage, and it's a great opportunity to get in a nice chunk of your hydration needs before the busyness of the day sets in. This is the one thing I've done every single day for the past seventeen-plus years. No matter where in the world I am, no matter what's going on in my life, the first thing I do is drink some water. I recommend drinking 16 to 30 ounces of water within the first 15 minutes after waking up. This is what constitutes taking your "inner bath." We generally take an outer bath or shower to get ourselves ready for the day, but isn't the inside more important?

While we are <u>asleep</u>, our bodies undertake hundreds of different <u>processes</u> to repair damaged tissues, fortify our <u>immune</u> system, eliminate old cells, and more.

No. 2   Have Some Mental Food

Legendary personal development teacher Zig Ziglar said, "People often say that motivation doesn't last. Well, neither does bathing—that's why we recommend it daily." This quote is a great pivot from taking an inner bath to pouring something into our spirit. Being that our mindset and perception determines our reality, there are few things more important than deciding the lens we're going to see life through to start the day. Taking 5 to 10 minutes to read, listen to, or watch something inspirational acts as mental food and a powerful reminder of how strong, capable, and amazing you really are. After having your morning water, tune into something empowering, like:

- Reading a selection from a thought-provoking book

- Listening to a selection from an inspiring audiobook or podcast

- Watching a short motivational video (there's nothing like watching a video from my friend Dr. Eric Thomas—aka ET The Hip-Hop Preacher—to put you in a dynamic state of mind!)

Another way to activate your inner power is through introspection. This could be through journaling, a gratitude practice, meditation, or whatever gets you tuned in to the person you want to be and what kind of day you're choosing to create. You can do a combination of any of these things, but it's ideal to select just *one* and truly make it a daily habit. No matter which one it is, make it a mandate to feed your mind to start your day.

No. 3 Move Your Body

This simple act will fortify your metabolic rate the rest of the day—and even improve your sleep quality at night. Most importantly, this doesn't have to be complicated! You don't need to do anything elaborate to extract these benefits. Doing something to elevate your heart rate and get your blood circulating for even 5 minutes can put you in a healthier metabolic state. Here are a few things you can place into your morning momentum routine:

- **A quick 5- to 10-minute power walk**
- **A short yoga session (a series of sun salutations fits nicely here)**
- **A few minutes of jumping rope**
- **A few minutes of jumping on a rebounder (aka a mini trampoline)**
- **A couple of circuits of body weight exercises**

The possibilities of ways to move our bodies are really endless. The vital thing is that we do *something* physical to get our day going. As mentioned, this can even help us sleep better at night because it helps to sync up our body's circadian rhythms. Appalachian State University conducted a study on morning, afternoon, and evening exercisers and found that morning exercisers have more efficient sleep cycles, they tend to sleep longer on average, and they spend more time in the deepest, most anabolic stages of sleep. This doesn't at all mean that you can't do your workout at other times of the day. But making sure to add in a little movement to start the day pays off bigger dividends when you lay your head down at night.[114]

No. 4 Eat When You're Ready

You don't have to cram down food to start the day if you don't want to. We were force-fed the narrative that "breakfast is the most important meal of the day" by the marketers of ultra-processed foods, not by science. In fact, the practice of Smart Intermittent Fasting that adheres to our body's natural circadian rhythms has been a part of human cultures for thousands of years.

Our body's circadian timing system is a network of interconnected cellular structures that regulate the timing of *all* physiological processes and behavior. Researchers at the Salk Institute for Biological Studies have uncovered that our circadian clocks are functional genes and proteins that influence and control other genes and proteins. And these clocks exist within each and every one of the trillions of cells within our bodies. The bottom line: Every one of our cells is synced up with the natural rhythms of the world around us. And we can align with that synchronicity, or we can take tiny hammers to those cellular clocks and smash them with our behaviors.[115]

A recent study published in the *British Journal of Nutrition* provides an eloquent description regarding circadian nutrition:

> The human circadian system anticipates and adapts to daily environmental changes to optimize behavior according to time of day and temporally partition incompatible physiological processes. At the helm of this system is a master clock in the suprachiasmatic nuclei (SCN) of the anterior hypothalamus. The SCN are primarily synchronized to the 24-hour day by the light/dark cycle; however, feeding/fasting cycles are the primary time cues for clocks in peripheral tissues. Aligning feeding/fasting cycles with clock-regulated metabolic changes optimizes metabolism, and studies of other animals suggest that feeding at inappropriate times disrupts circadian system organization and thereby contributes to adverse metabolic consequences and chronic disease development.[116]

The question then arises: If eating at inappropriate times disrupts our metabolic system, when are the ideal times to eat? The most important thing to remember is that this is going to vary from person to person because we are all unique. But there are a few consistent things to take note of to give us the greatest metabolic advantage.

According to a study published in the journal *Cell Metabolism*, the average person is eating through the span of about 15 hours a day **(the time between the first bite of breakfast and the last bite of dinner or an evening snack)**, which is nearly the entire time most people are awake. The scientists in the study decided to see what would happen if they simply shortened the window of eating for some of the test subjects. **There was no other dietary advice given—no restriction on calories, food choices, macronutrient ratios, or anything else.** They simply had study participants reduce their eating to a period of 10 to 12 hours a day instead of the sporadic 15 hours a day that was typical, and here's what happened: After sixteen weeks, without any standard dietary restriction, by shortening their eating window by a few hours, the study participants lost an average of over 7 pounds. The study volunteers also subjectively reported that they were sleeping better and having a lot more energy. An analysis of their diets also uncovered that they'd naturally reduced their calorie intake by about 20 percent (even though there were no calorie restrictions placed on them). They were losing weight, eating foods they enjoyed, and experiencing a lot more energy. It might sound too good to be true on the surface, but there's a lot more going on behind the scenes.[117]

One of the most remarkable things about Smart Intermittent Fasting is that it initiates hormonal changes that make stored body fat more accessible. Data published in the peer-reviewed journal *Obesity* states that employing intermittent fasting is like flipping a "metabolic switch" that shifts the metabolism from fat creation and fat storage to mobilization of body fat in the form of free fatty acids and fatty acid–derived ketones to be used for fuel.[118]

Another study conducted by researchers at the University of Copenhagen found that intermittent fasting is able to quickly reduce insulin resistance and nullify the effects of insulin-created roadblocks that stop fat from being released from the cells. Their study also revealed that intermittent fasting has some significant effects on our vital satiety hormones.[119]

Research published in the journal *Endocrinology* reports that intermittent fasting can improve the function of satiety-related hormones like neuropeptide Y, while supporting fat loss and retaining lean muscle mass. A startling percentage of people who lose weight through conventional calorie restriction regain their lost fat and find it exceedingly harder to lose weight over time. A huge player in this metabolic conundrum is a loss of their body's valuable muscle mass.[120]

Now, here's the thing...you do not have to jump through a bunch of hoops to extract some of these benefits and get your body's clock set to a healthy rhythm. In the aforementioned study cited in *Obesity*, the researchers stated that the metabolic switch typically occurs 12-plus hours after cessation of food consumption. Plus, a study published in the journal *Annals of Nutrition and Metabolism* showed that a daily 12-hour intermittent fast was enough to significantly reduce levels of homocysteine and C-reactive protein, which are both major markers of heart disease and systemic inflammation. Simply finishing your last meal of the day by 8:00 p.m., hanging out for a bit and getting a good night's rest, then having your first food after 8:00 a.m. the next morning is an easy example of kick-starting these benefits. Smart intermittent fasting is about feeling good and doing what works best for *you*.[121]

Just follow these four simple steps:

F Figure out your ideal eating and fasting windows.

A Adjust your windows to fit your lifestyle.

S Safeguard with supportive nutrition.

T Track how you look, feel, and perform.

A little intention in your daily eating routine can go a long way. Here are a couple of sample routines you can follow:

Standard Eat Smarter Format

with 12-HOUR EATING WINDOW

Time	
Midnight	Sleeping and/or Fasting
4 a.m.	
8 a.m.	Eating
Noon	
4 p.m.	
8 p.m.	Sleeping and/or Fasting
Midnight	

Smart Intermittent Fasting Format I

with 10-HOUR EATING WINDOW

Time	
Midnight	Sleeping and/or Fasting
4 a.m.	
10 a.m.	Eating
Noon	
4 p.m.	
8 p.m.	Sleeping and/or Fasting
Midnight	

Smart Intermittent Fasting Format II

with 8-HOUR EATING WINDOW

Time	
Midnight	Sleeping and/or Fasting
4 a.m.	
10 a.m.	
Noon	Eating
4 p.m.	
8 p.m.	Sleeping and/or Fasting
Midnight	

No. 5 Sip Some Supportive Nutrition

Since you can "break" your overnight fast whenever you want (by having your first meal), in the meantime and in-between time having some supportive nutrition can help take things to another level.

After drinking water, getting in some mental nourishment, and doing a little exercise, I always make my wife and myself some coffee or tea, and I make my youngest son his favorite hot cacao drink whenever he has a day off from school. We covered some of the remarkable benefits of coffee and tea earlier in Chapter Three. But one of the best times to gather these benefits is in a fasted state in the morning.

In addition to the metabolic and cognitive benefits we already covered, a study published in the *American Journal of Clinical Nutrition* revealed that coffee is an excellent adjunct during a fasting window because it helps stimulate a variety of satiety hormones, including cholecystokinin (CCK). Produced primarily by cells in the gut, CCK is a prolific hormone that plays a role in many aspects of fat metabolism. Plus, one of the nutrients found in coffee called chlorogenic acid has been found to increase the breakdown of stored fat while increasing protection of muscle tissue. Anything that helps to maintain your valuable muscle tissue is especially valuable. Coffee—without all of the typical additives like conventional sugar and creamers laced with artificial sweeteners, or pesticides—can support your health in a variety of ways. We'll be able to take those benefits up a few notches with the Superhero Coffee recipe in the Drinks & Smoothies chapter. Additionally, our Chai with Ghee, B's Hot Cocoa (which kids love), or a simple cup of green tea are a great way to start your day and provide your body with a wealth of phenomenal nutrients.[122,123]

Now It's Time to Eat!

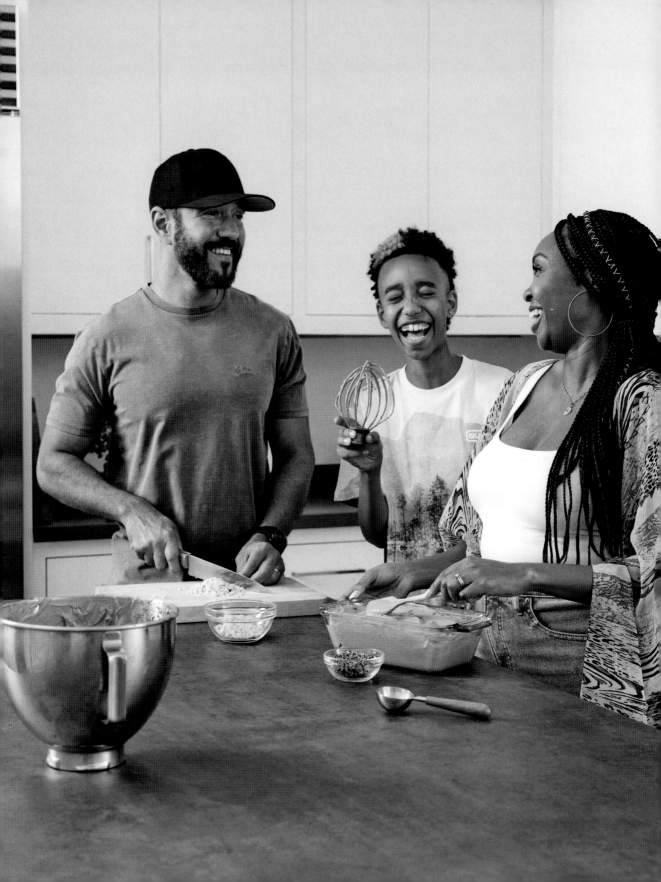

Sample Family Meal Plan

	Monday	**Tuesday**	**Wednesday** Optional Meal Prep Day
Meal One	Southwest Chorizo Scramble (page 117)	Leftovers	Turkey Bacon Breakfast Burritos (page 131)
Meal Two Or Snack	Speedy Superfood Guacamole (page 244) + veggie slices	Açai Protein Bowl (page 118)	Leftovers
Meal Three	Supreme Salmon Burgers (page 187) + Better Brussels Sprouts (page 235)	Stuffed Sweet Potatoes (page 213) + Steamed Broccoli with Grass-Fed Butter (page 225)	Slow Cooker Chicken Curry (page 194) + Mushroom Fried Rice (page 233)
Optional Snack	Superfood Chocolate Bark (page 260)	Smoky Spicy Mixed Nuts (page 247)	Cashew Butter Planets (page 255)

Thursday	Friday	Saturday	Sunday
			Optional Meal Prep Day
Spicy Protein Breakfast Bowl (page 121)	Power Protein Omelet (page 122) + Kimchi	Sweet Potato Protein Pancakes (page 127)	Bacon, Spinach, & Bell Pepper Quiche (page 134)
Faux Salmon Nori Wraps (page 179) + kimchi	Superfood Salad (page 160)	Leftovers	PB&J Superfood Shake (page 153)
Leftovers	Honey Sriracha Salmon (page 193) + Easy Quinoa and Cauliflower "Pilaf" (page 234)	Buffalo Chicken Tacos (page 221)	Southwest BBQ Chicken Salad (page 159)
Quick and Easy Deviled Eggs (page 250)	Cherry Frozen Yogurt Pops (page 269)	Smarter Snickers Bites (page 262)	Pumpkin Muffins (page 257)

Note: It's essential to begin each day with proper hydration and to ensure you're hitting your hydration target throughout the day. As noted previously, the metabolic and cognitive benefits it provides is unmatched.

Additionally, if you're utilizing Smart Intermittent Fasting, having some Superhero Coffee, Chai with Ghee, or simply some green or herbal tea can carry over and replace the need/desire for one of your meals. It's totally up to you! Just ensure that you are eating adequate protein and getting in plenty of micronutrients when you do have your meals.

Breakfast

CHAPTER FOUR   The *Eat Smarter Family Cookbook* is based on scientific data and lots of deliciousness! From a scientific perspective, your first meal of the day literally sets the tone for your metabolic health. Researchers at the University of Kansas Medical Center used fMRIs and discovered that adding in more protein, specifically for your first meal of the day, decreases the signals in the brain that stimulate appetite and lead to overeating. A performance like this should be making front page news! Luckily, you have this information in your hands. These tasty breakfast dishes are designed to provide the ample amount of protein your body needs to thrive. Keep in mind, although they get the breakfast tag, these delicious meals can be eaten at any time of the day.[1]

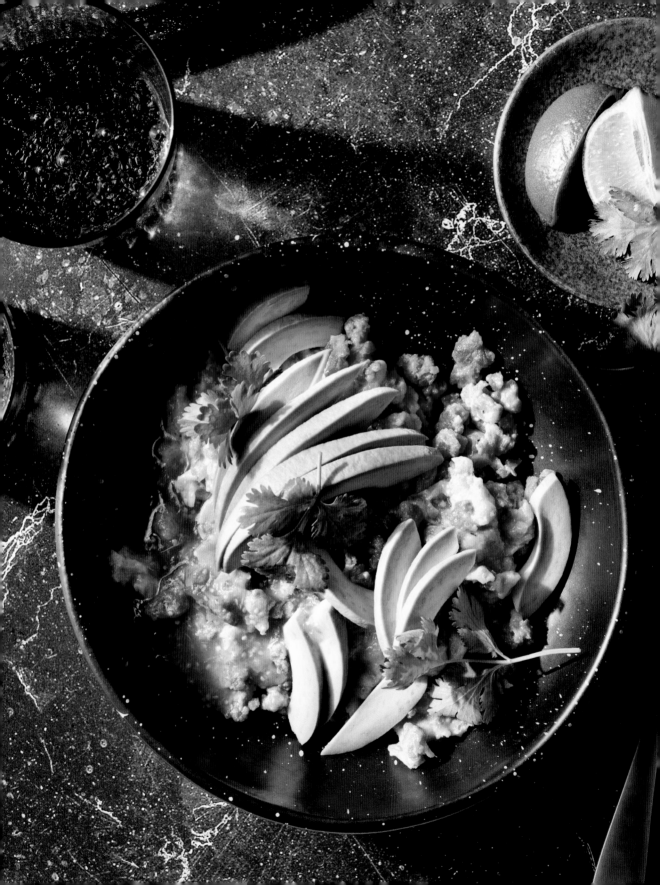

Southwest Chorizo Scramble

Breakfast scrambles are a great way to add a diversity of macro- and micronutrients to your diet. This Southwest-style scramble is super tasty, easy to make, and packed with ingredients that support cognition and metabolic health. For variety, you can add anything you have on hand to this scramble (that's what makes scrambles so awesome!). Mushrooms, sweet peppers, hot peppers, spinach, onions—the list goes on and on.

Heat a sauté pan over medium heat. Add the chorizo and cook, breaking it up with a wooden spoon or spatula, until lightly browned and cooked through, 2 to 3 minutes.

Crack the eggs into a mixing bowl, whisk together with the turmeric, and season lightly with salt and pepper. Add the eggs to the pan and cook, scrambling with a wooden spoon or spatula, until the eggs are cooked to your preference. Transfer the scramble to two plates and top with salsa and avocado slices. Enjoy.

Serves 2

¼ pound ground chorizo

4 large organic eggs

¼ teaspoon ground turmeric

Sea salt and black pepper

¼ cup salsa of your choice

1 ripe large avocado, peeled, pitted, and sliced

Açai Protein Bowl

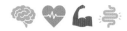

Açai bowls are a family favorite. Being that I'm a bona fide blender chef, I love making these delicious bowls when I have friends over as well. It gets grown people and kids alike scraping the bottom of the bowl (and I've even caught people using their finger) to get every morsel of açai they possibly can. Please note, since we are using frozen packets, you may need to thaw them a tiny bit to cut them open but do not, I repeat, do not unfreeze them too much! They need to be as frozen as possible when you add them to the blender to maintain the ice cream consistency you want. We intentionally want to keep the liquid ingredients to a minimum. Thus, only a couple of tablespoons of almond milk. This means you'll be using a tamper/pushing tool to push the ingredients around and towards the blades while blending.

Add the açai berries, banana, blueberries, nut butter, flaxseeds, honey, whey protein, and almond milk to a high-speed blender (see Note). Blend, using a tamper to keep the ingredients moving around and catching in the blade, until you reach an ice cream/sorbet consistency.

Divide the mixture between two bowls and add toppings of choice. The sky's the limit of deliciousness here.

Note: This recipe requires a high-speed blender (Vitamix, Blendtec, etc.) for the best ice cream–like consistency.

Serves 2

- **2 (100g) packets frozen organic 100% açai berries (nothing else added)**
- **1 frozen peeled banana, cut in chunks**
- **¾ cup frozen blueberries**
- **2 tablespoons salted sugar-free peanut or almond butter**
- **3 tablespoons ground flaxseeds**
- **1 tablespoon raw honey**
- **2 scoops (about ⅔ cup) vanilla or chocolate whey protein or plant-based protein powder (at least 20g protein per serving)**
- **2 tablespoons unsweetened almond milk**

SUGGESTED TOPPINGS

- **Diced banana**
- **Crushed walnuts**
- **Extra peanut or almond butter**
- **Organic granola**
- **Sliced strawberries**
- **Cacao nibs**
- **Extra raw honey**

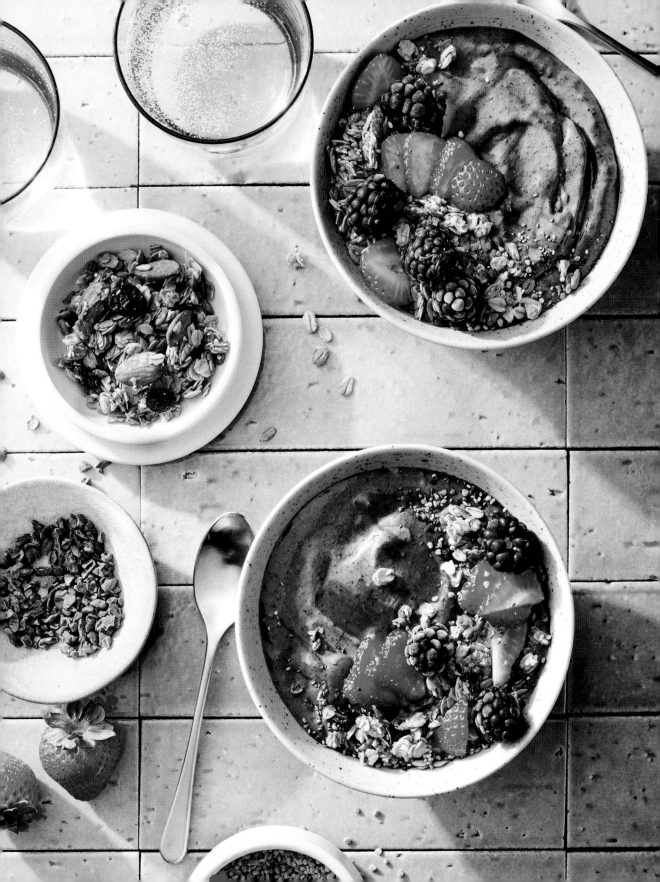

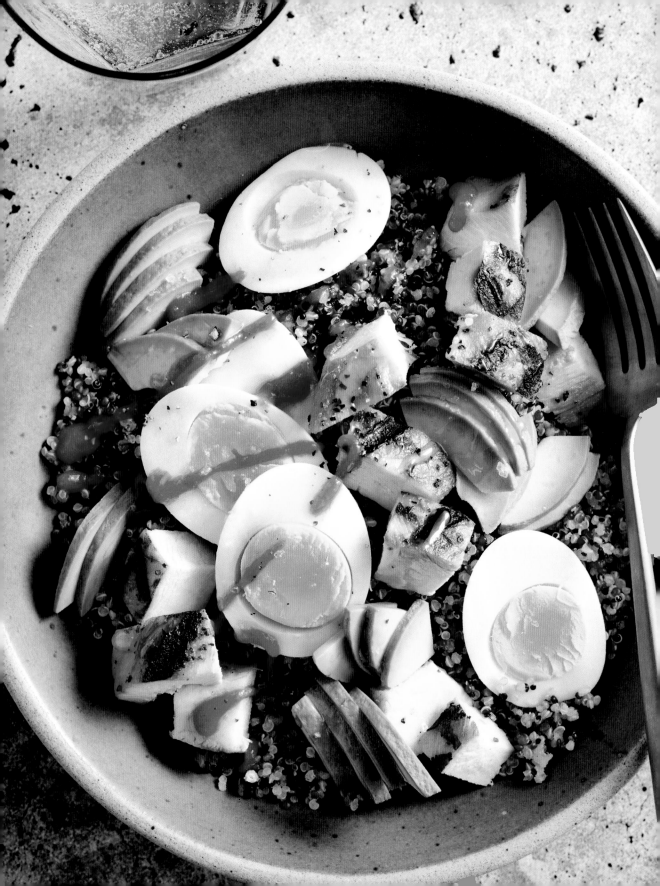

Spicy Protein Breakfast Bowl

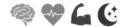

Power-packed with protein, this spicy breakfast bowl is great for any time of the day! This is a great way to use up leftover grains—I use quinoa here but brown rice or farro would also be delicious. This recipe includes chicken breast, but you could instead utilize boneless skinless baked chicken thighs or even store-bought rotisserie chicken.

Divide the quinoa between two bowls. Add 1½ eggs along with ¾ cup of the chicken to each bowl. Top with avocado slices, then drizzle with the sriracha and honey. Serve and enjoy!

Serves 2

- **1½ cups cooked quinoa (preferably cooked in bone broth, but water is fine)**
- **3 hard-boiled large organic eggs, peeled and sliced**
- **1½ cups diced leftover cooked, seasoned chicken breast**
- **1 ripe large avocado, pitted, peeled, and sliced**
- **4 teaspoons sriracha hot sauce**
- **2 teaspoons raw honey**

Protein Power Omelet

Omelets are a classic breakfast item that enable us to gracefully mix in veggies with plenty of high-powered protein. The smarter additions like the turmeric and miso mayo add amazing flavor notes, plus bonus cognitive and metabolic benefits. You'll have to hold yourself back from saying, "Omelet you feel these gains!" after adding dishes like this to your repertoire. For variety, you can add diced portobello mushrooms, tomato, scallions, jalapeños, or any other veggies you enjoy. Serve with a side of fermented veggies like sauerkraut or kimchi.

Crack the eggs into a mixing bowl and whisk to combine. Add the spinach, turmeric, salt, and pepper to the bowl and whisk again.

Heat the coconut oil in a safe nonstick skillet or well-seasoned cast-iron pan over medium-low heat. When the pan is warm, pour in the egg mixture and let it sit for a minute or so to set up. Continue cooking the omelet, using a wooden spoon or spatula to gently pull in the edges, tilting the pan to fill them in with raw egg mixture from the center, until the bottom is set and the top is almost cooked through. (This should take 2 to 3 minutes.)

Sprinkle on the shredded cheese and diced meat and fold the omelet over.

Plate the omelet and add the spicy mayo and avocado slices on top.

Serves 1

3 large organic eggs

½ cup thinly sliced spinach

¼ cup shredded cheese of your choice (about 1 ounce)

¼ teaspoon ground turmeric

⅛ teaspoon fine sea salt

⅛ teaspoon black pepper

1½ teaspoons coconut oil

¼ cup diced ham or cooked sausage, or crumbled cooked bacon

1 tablespoon Miso Mayo (page 281)

½ ripe avocado, pitted, peeled, and thinly sliced

Sweet Potato and Pepper Hash with Avocado

Sweet potatoes have been absolutely booming at the culinary box office. Though they've been prized for thousands of years, sweet potatoes have recently stepped in to sub for white potatoes in a way that's reminiscent of Kevin Feige stepping in and taking Marvel Studios from "meh" to a multigenerational megastar. Sweet potato versions of everything from fries to chips to casseroles are all pretty popular now. But one of my ultimate favorites is this sweet potato hash. It's an excellent choice for breakfast, and it also makes a delicious dinner, too. Feel free to mix it up with the other veggies. And if you prefer over-easy or poached eggs, just cook the hash and eggs separately.

Bring a pot of salted water up to a boil. Add sweet potato and cook for 10 to 12 minutes, until tender when pierced with a knife. Drain and set aside.

Heat 2 tablespoons of the oil in a 9- or 10-inch safe nonstick sauté pan or well-seasoned cast-iron pan over medium heat. Add the onion and bell pepper, and season with salt and pepper. Cook for 3 to 5 minutes, until the onions are translucent and the peppers are starting to brown.

Add 1 more tablespoon of the oil, the sweet potato, the garlic powder, cumin, and ground chipotle and cook for another 5 to 8 minutes, until the sweet potato browns in places, trying not to stir too much.

Make four little wells in the hash, fill each with a little less than a teaspoon of the remaining oil, and crack in the eggs. Turn the heat down to medium-low, season with salt and pepper, cover with a lid (it can be from another pot or pan, just try to find one that fits) and cook for 4 to 6 minutes, until the whites are set but the yolks are still runny. (Cook longer if you prefer your eggs more well-done.) Transfer to serving plates and garnish with sliced avocado and cilantro. Serve lime wedges on the side.

Serves 2 to 4

- **2 small to medium or 1 large sweet potato, peeled and cut into ½-inch dice**
- **4 tablespoons avocado oil**
- **½ small red onion, diced (about ½ cup)**
- **1 red bell pepper, cored, seeded, and diced**
- **Sea salt and black pepper**
- **½ teaspoon garlic powder**
- **½ teaspoon ground cumin**
- **Pinch of ground chipotle, or to taste**
- **4 large organic eggs**
- **1 ripe avocado, pitted, peeled, and sliced**
- **¼ cup chopped fresh cilantro leaves**
- **Lime wedges**

Upgraded Breakfast Sandwich

I always loved breakfast sandwiches when I was a kid. There's a great scene in the movie *Big Daddy* starring Adam Sandler where he hustles to get his kid to McDonald's before 11:00 a.m. to get breakfast (including a breakfast sandwich for a homeless fella they met along the way–played by Steve Buscemi), only to find out that they actually stopped serving breakfast at 10:30 a.m. Comedy ensues from top to bottom, but I could always identify with rushing to McDonald's before the sacred cutoff time hit and eggs were no longer allowed. I wanted to find a way to upgrade the classic breakfast sandwich for my kids, and this one is definitely a hit!

Heat a large frying pan over medium-high heat. Add the sausage patties and cook, flipping once, until the meat is nicely browned and cooked through. Set aside on a large plate. Pour the grease into the trash and wipe out the pan.

Heat the pan over medium heat, add 1 tablespoon butter, and spread it around evenly. Crack the eggs into the pan and season with salt and pepper. Break the yolks and fry the eggs until they're firm enough to flip. Flip the eggs and fry until cooked through. Transfer the eggs to the plate while you prepare the rest of the sandwich.

Coat the pan with the oil spray, or melt the extra butter and swirl in the cayenne. Add the bread and cook for about 30 seconds per side, just long enough to give it a little color and firmness. Place 1 slice of bread on each serving plate and top with 2 fried eggs, a sausage patty, and half of the avocado slices. Coat the top slices of bread with fruit spread and place on the sandwich. Cut in half and enjoy!

Serves 2

- 2 sandwich-sized sausage patties
- 1 tablespoon salted grass-fed butter
- 4 large organic eggs
- Sea salt and black pepper
- Chipotle-infused avocado oil spray, or coconut oil cooking spray or 2 extra tablespoons grass-fed butter plus a large pinch of cayenne pepper (see Note)
- 4 slices sourdough bread
- ½ ripe avocado, pitted, peeled, and sliced
- 2 tablespoons organic fruit spread with no added sugar (strawberry or grape are ideal)

Note: One of the upgrades to classic breakfast sandwiches is the sourdough bread. Sourdough's use dates back to 2000 BC by the ancient Egyptians, and several other cultures prior to that. They knew it was an ideal way to improve the nutrient profile and reduce the presence of antinutrients. An alternative would be to use a sprouted grain bread, but sourdough works great here.

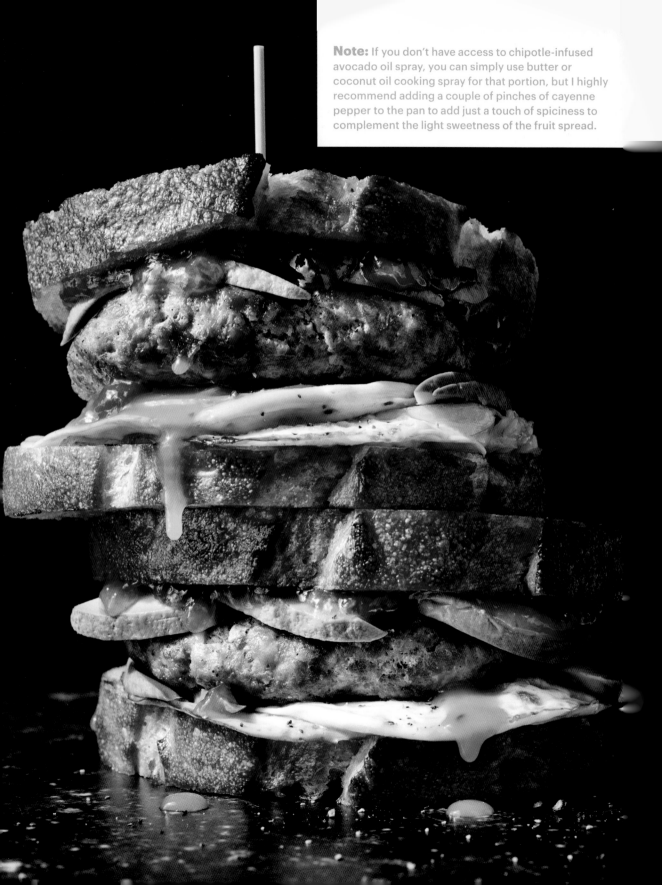

Note: If you don't have access to chipotle-infused avocado oil spray, you can simply use butter or coconut oil cooking spray for that portion, but I highly recommend adding a couple of pinches of cayenne pepper to the pan to add just a touch of spiciness to complement the light sweetness of the fruit spread.

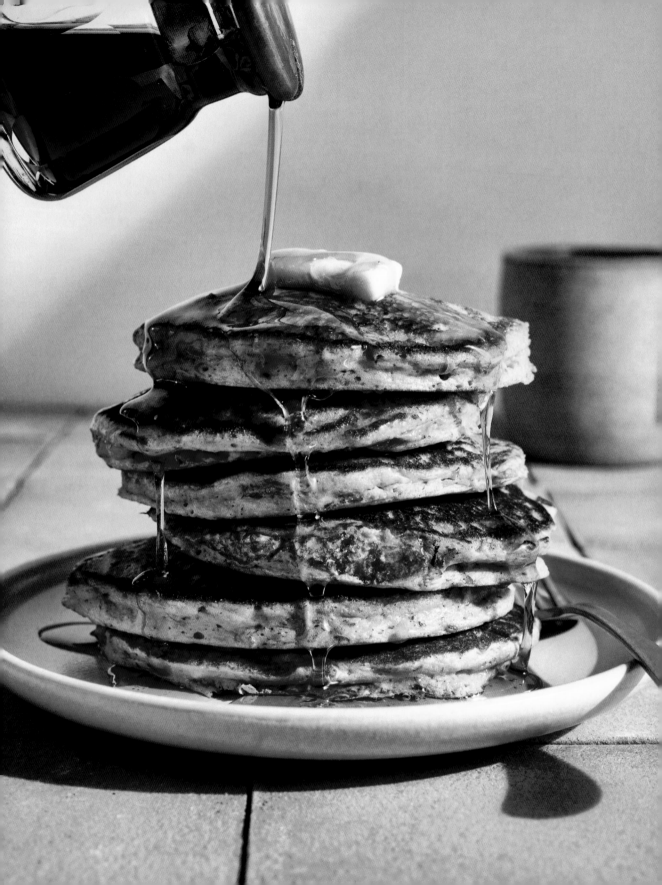

Sweet Potato Protein Pancakes

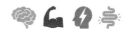

Pancakes are synonymous with breakfast today. But what if we could transform typical pancakes that leave you feeling flat into scrumptious, protein-packed pancakes that have you feeling satisfied and strong? That's what this recipe delivers. Serve them hot out of the pan with your favorite toppings, or make a big batch to freeze for a quick reheat-and-go breakfast through the week. Keep in mind, these are not your typical run-of-the-mill pancakes. These are packed with real-food ingredients that support your microbiome and metabolism.

Preheat the oven to 400°F. Prick the sweet potatoes all over with a fork and roast for 1 hour or until very tender. Remove from the oven and let cool.

When the sweet potatoes are cool enough to handle, remove the skin. Measure out 2 cups cooked flesh and transfer to a large mixing bowl. Use an electric hand mixer or potato masher to mix until smooth.

Whisk in the eggs, almond milk, and vanilla extract to combine. Add the flaxseeds, cassava flour, salt, baking powder, and protein powder and mix well. Let the batter sit for a minute or two while you heat a large, safe nonstick skillet or frying pan over medium heat. Add some oil and slowly pour or scoop the batter in, using approximately ¼ cup for each pancake.

Cook the pancakes for 2 to 3 minutes per side, then transfer to a plate or platter. Repeat in batches, adding oil to the pan as needed.

Serve with butter and maple syrup or your toppings of choice!

Serves 4 to 6

- **2 medium-to-large sweet potatoes**
- **4 large organic eggs**
- **¼ cup unsweetened almond milk**
- **1 teaspoon vanilla extract**
- **2 tablespoons ground flaxseeds**
- **2 tablespoons cassava flour**
- **¼ teaspoon kosher salt**
- **2 teaspoons baking powder**
- **2 scoops (about ⅔ cup) vanilla protein powder (40g protein total)**
- **Coconut oil**
- **Salted grass-fed butter and maple syrup or other toppings**

Asparagus and Olive Frittata

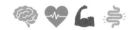

This delicious, colorful frittata is one of my favorites. Anytime I can add in some olives, I'm a happier man. When I was a kid, I was only familiar with the creepy pimento-stuffed olives my mom used to buy that looked like a jar of alien eyes. Thankfully, I've now had the opportunity to try countless varieties of olives and I understand why humans have been writing about them adoringly for centuries. Be sure to use a well-seasoned cast-iron pan or safe nonstick pan for this so your frittata is easy to remove and serve.

Preheat the oven to 375°F.

Heat 2 tablespoons of the olive oil in a 9- or 10-inch safe nonstick sauté pan or well-seasoned cast-iron pan over medium heat. Add the asparagus and scallions, season with salt and pepper, and sauté for 3 to 5 minutes, until the asparagus are lightly cooked through. Stir in the spinach and cook for another 2 minutes, until wilted. Turn off the heat.

Crack the eggs into a large mixing bowl and whisk together with ¾ teaspoon salt and ¼ teaspoon pepper. Mix in the olives, feta, and parsley, then stir in the cooked vegetables.

Give the pan a wipe if there are any bits left behind, then place it over medium heat. Add the remaining 2 tablespoons oil and pour in the frittata mixture. Cook for about 1 minute, until the edges are just starting to brown.

Transfer to the oven and cook for about 20 minutes, until the eggs are completely cooked through.

Let cool for at least 5 minutes before slicing and serving.

Note: Feta is great here, but soft goat cheese or even grated parmesan would also be delicious.

Serves 4 to 6

- **4 tablespoons olive oil**
- **½ bunch asparagus, woody ends removed, cut into ½-inch pieces (about 2 cups)**
- **6 scallions or 1 small leek (white and light green parts), thinly sliced**
- **Kosher salt and black pepper**
- **2 cups packed baby spinach, roughly chopped**
- **8 large organic eggs**
- **¼ cup roughly chopped pitted kalamata olives**
- **½ cup crumbled feta cheese (about 4 ounces; see Note)**
- **3 tablespoons chopped fresh parsley**

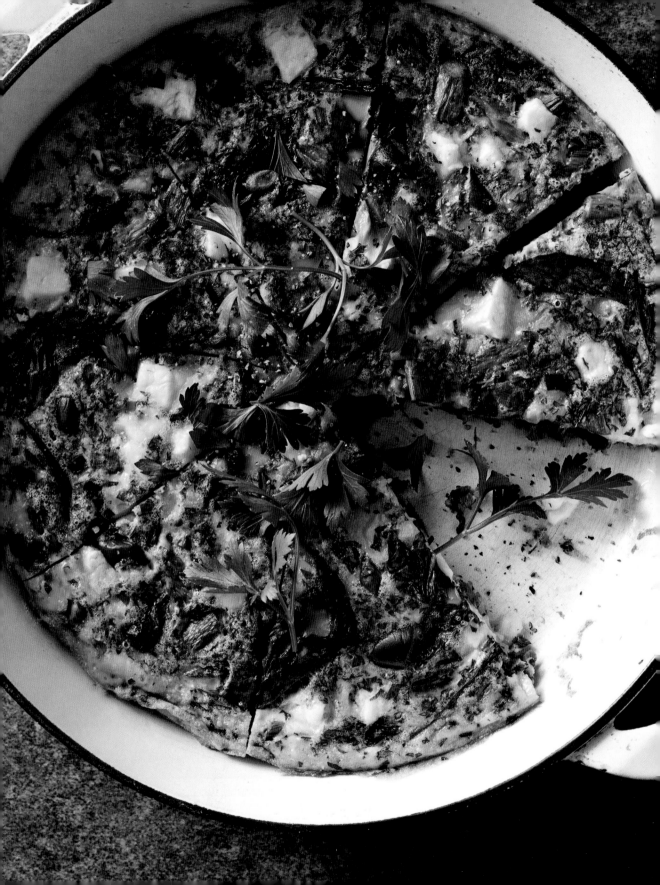

Bacon and Veggie Egg Cups

This is a staple grab-and-go breakfast at our house. It's a great way to jam-pack real-food nutrition into fun little muffin shapes. Your family can have them fresh out of the oven, or you can whip them up and store them in the fridge to reheat and eat whenever you desire. It's also super versatile, so you can mix and match veggies and meats in any way you want!

Preheat the oven to 375°F.

Put the bacon, broccoli, and mushrooms on a large baking sheet and toss with the avocado oil and garlic powder. Season generously with salt and pepper. Make sure that the ingredients are spread out and not overlapping, so they can start to brown in the oven. Roast for 12 to 15 minutes, until the bacon is beginning to crisp up and the veggies are tender. Remove from the oven and turn the heat down to 350°F.

Meanwhile, crack the eggs into a large mixing bowl and whisk together with ½ teaspoon salt and ¼ teaspoon pepper.

Put 12 paper liners in a muffin tray and divide the baby spinach between them. Sprinkle over the grated cheese, then divide the bacon, mushrooms, and broccoli between the cups. Carefully pour over the egg mixture. (You want the cups to be about three-quarters full.) Top each one with a little more grated cheese, if you like. Transfer to the oven and bake for 25 to 28 minutes, until puffed and lightly golden. Remove from the oven and allow them to cool. Serve or store for later.

Makes 12 cups

4 slices bacon, finely diced

1 cup finely chopped broccoli florets

1 cup sliced cremini mushrooms

1 teaspoon avocado oil

½ teaspoon garlic powder

Kosher salt and black pepper

10 large organic eggs

1 cup packed baby spinach or arugula, finely chopped

½ cup grated cheese such as cheddar or parmesan, plus extra if desired

Turkey Bacon Breakfast Burritos

These breakfast burritos are like a tortilla decided to give a big, loving hug to a bunch of delicious meats, veggies, and healthy fats. They're great for weekly meal prep as they keep well in the refrigerator for a few days—and freeze well, too. The tortilla is your prerogative. It can be any type of large tortilla—spinach, sprouted grain, coconut, or almond flour are all great options!

Heat 1 tablespoon of the oil in a large sauté pan over medium-high heat. Add the bacon and cook for 5 to 8 minutes, until it is starting to brown and get crispy around the edges.

Add the remaining tablespoon oil and the broccoli, bell pepper, and onion. Season with salt and pepper and cook, stirring often, for 5 minutes or until the broccoli is just tender.

Meanwhile, crack the eggs into a medium mixing bowl. Season with ½ teaspoon salt and ¼ teaspoon pepper, and whisk to combine. Taste the bacon-veggie mixture for seasoning and add more salt and/or pepper if desired. Pour in the eggs. Turn the heat down to medium-low and cook for about 3 minutes, stirring often, until the eggs are cooked through. (You want them on the firm side so your burrito isn't too wet.) Stir in the cheese and transfer the mixture to a large plate to cool slightly.

Clean out the pan and put it back over medium heat. Working one at a time, heat a tortilla, transfer it to a cutting board, and top with one-quarter of the egg mixture. Arrange one-quarter of the avocado slices down the center, if using, and carefully roll it into a tight burrito, starting at the bottom and folding in the sides as you roll. If you like a seared or sealed-shut burrito, add it back into the hot pan, seam side down, for 5 to 10 seconds. Serve with your favorite hot sauce or salsa on the side.

Serves 4

- **2 tablespoons avocado oil**
- **4 slices turkey bacon, diced**
- **1½ cups finely chopped broccoli florets**
- **½ red bell pepper, seeded and diced**
- **¼ small white onion, finely diced (about ⅓ cup)**
- **Kosher salt and black pepper**
- **8 large organic eggs**
- **½ cup grated cheese (such as cheddar)**
- **4 burrito-sized tortillas (see headnote)**
- **1 ripe avocado, pitted, peeled, and thinly sliced (optional)**
- **Hot sauce or salsa**

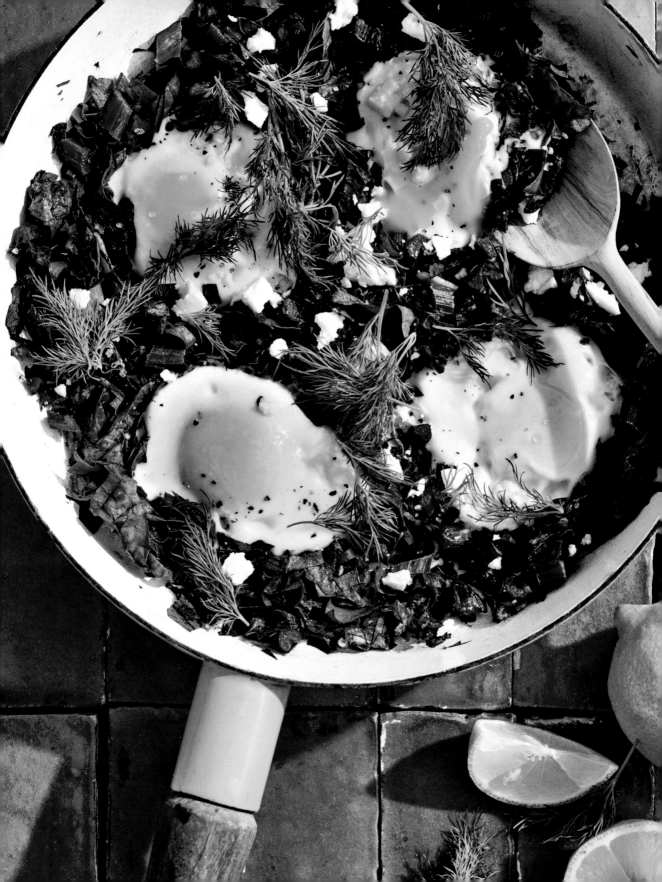

Swiss Chard Egg Nests with Feta, Dill, and Lemon

In Chapter Three, we covered a study from researchers at Chicago's Rush University Medical Center that found that people who ate one to two servings of leafy greens each day experienced fewer memory problems and less cognitive decline than folks who didn't reach that benchmark. A great way to ensure that we hit that target is to get in a serving or two during that first meal of the day. This recipe satisfies that goal *and* satisfies the taste buds.

Heat 2 tablespoons of the olive oil in a 9- or 10-inch safe nonstick sauté pan or well-seasoned cast-iron pan over medium heat. Add garlic and cook for about 30 seconds, until fragrant and just starting to brown around the edges. Add the chard and a good pinch of salt, and sauté for another 5 minutes or until the chard is wilted.

Make four wells in the chard. Fill each well with just under a teaspoon of the remaining olive oil and crack in 1 egg. Season with salt and pepper, cover with a lid (it can be from another pot or pan; just try to find one that fits), and cook over medium-low heat for 4 to 6 minutes, until the whites are just set.

Transfer to plates and garnish with the feta and the dill, if using. Serve with lemon wedges on the side.

Serves 2

3 tablespoons olive oil

3 garlic cloves, thinly sliced

1 bunch red Swiss chard, stems included, roughly chopped (about 5 cups packed)

Sea salt and black pepper

4 large organic eggs

¼ cup crumbled feta cheese

2 tablespoons chopped fresh dill (optional)

Lemon wedges

Bacon, Spinach, and Bell Pepper Quiche

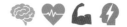

My family loves this recipe so much that we'll often make it when we have guests over for brunch. Little do they know, whenever I hear the word "quiche" I can't help but think of the scene from the movie *White Men Can't Jump* when Rosie Perez's character is living her dream as a contestant on the game show *Jeopardy!*. She confidently tore through the category of *Foods that start with the letter "Q"* and when I heard her say "quiche" for one of the answers, it was immortalized in my mind. It wasn't until two decades later that I had my first slice of a quiche. And it was so good that I went back for a Daily Double.

Preheat the oven to 350°F. Coat a 9-inch round pie plate with cooking spray.

To make the crust, mix together the almond flour, egg, coconut oil, and salt in a bowl with a spatula or wooden spoon until fully combined. Press the dough into the pie plate, pushing it evenly up the sides. Bake for 13 to 15 minutes, until the crust is lightly golden. Remove the crust from the oven, but leave the oven on.

Meanwhile, fry the bacon in a large skillet over medium heat until crisp. Transfer to a paper towel–lined plate. Pour out most of the bacon fat and add the bell peppers to the pan. Sauté until tender, 5 to 7 minutes.

Crack the eggs into a medium mixing bowl. Add the cream, salt, pepper, and onion powder and whisk to combine. Set aside.

Place the pie plate on a baking sheet. Transfer the peppers to the baked crust and top with the spinach. Chop or crumble the cooked bacon and sprinkle it over the spinach. Top with the cheese. Pour over the custard mixture, pressing down the filling ingredients to make sure they are submerged. Bake for 35 to 38 minutes, until the top is lightly golden, and the eggs are set. Cool for at least 15 minutes before slicing.

Serves 6

CRUST

Cooking spray

2 tablespoons coconut oil, melted

2 cups almond flour

1 large organic egg

1 teaspoon kosher salt

FILLING

4 slices bacon

2 red bell peppers, cored, seeded, and thinly sliced

¾ cup lightly packed baby spinach, thinly sliced

¾ cup grated cheddar or Gruyère cheese

3 large organic eggs

1 cup heavy cream

¼ teaspoon kosher salt

¼ teaspoon black pepper

1 teaspoon onion powder

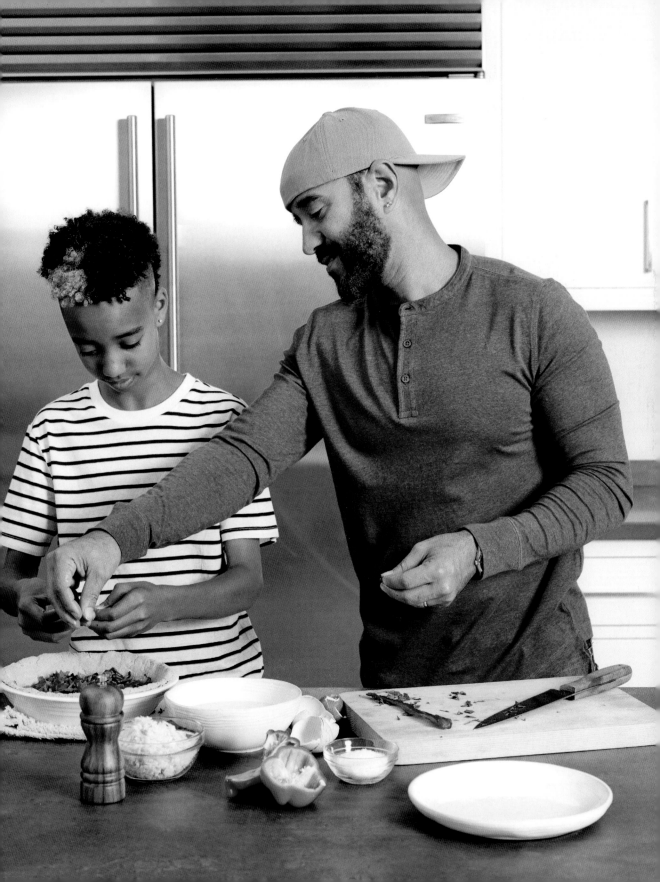

Drinks & Smoothies

CHAPTER FIVE These drinks and smoothies are designed to deliver some serious nutrition plus some serious enjoyment. Based on the results you want, they can be a great way to jump-start your day, fuel your brain for high performance, or help you recover and re-energize after a workout.

Superhero Coffee

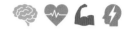

About ten years ago I came across a video from my friend Daniel Vitalis where he was making an "elixir," combining ingredients that blew my mind. He was using teas and herbs I was familiar with, like reishi and chaga, but he said your tea can become a "meal" by adding high-quality fats to it. It should have been obvious, since folks have been adding milk and cream to tea and coffee for centuries, but it opened my eyes to adding things like coconut oil, grass-fed butter, ghee, and nut milks like cashew or almond. Plus, I love a coffee that is infused with other potent brain- and metabolism-boosting ingredients like medicinal mushrooms. As you've discovered in the earlier chapters, the *quality* of your coffee matters a lot! I have a list of my favorite sources of coffees and teas for you in the bonus resources guide at eatsmartercookbook.com/bonus.

Combine the coffee, butter, MCT oil, lion's mane and stevia (if using), and cinnamon in your favorite coffee cup and blend with an electric hand mixer or frother, or combine in a blender and blend for 5 to 10 seconds.

Note: Instead of coffee, you can easily use tea in this recipe. Yerba mate, black tea, and rooibos are all great options. And if you want a boost of peptide support for your skin, bones, and joints, try adding 10g of collagen peptides (about a tablespoon).

Serves 1

- **1 cup hot, fresh brewed organic coffee (ideally infused with medicinal mushrooms like chaga and/or lion's mane; see Note)**
- **1 tablespoon salted grass-fed butter or ghee**
- **1 tablespoon MCT oil**
- **½ teaspoon lion's mane medicinal mushroom powder (optional; if you don't have a coffee blend that comes with it already)**
- **5 to 8 drops flavored stevia (chocolate or English toffee are good choices; optional)**
- **A few pinches of ground organic cinnamon**

Smarter Green Smoothie

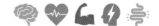

A meta-analysis published in the journal *Nutrients* uncovered that people who eat more than four servings of vegetables per day have the lowest risk for excess weight gain compared to those who undershoot this guideline. A green smoothie is an excellent way to get a jump start on your veggie intake to start the day. The Smarter Green Smoothie is my go-to recipe, but there are so many awesome variations you can make to diversify your nutrient intake. For instance, instead of spinach you can sub in kale or romaine lettuce. You can also swap out peanut butter for cashew or almond butter. One thing I highly recommend is adding in a serving of a superfood "greens" blend for an additional burst of micronutrients. I have a few of my favorites for you in the bonus resources guide at eatsmartercookbook.com/bonus.[2]

Combine the banana, spinach, blueberries, protein powder, nut butter, almond milk, and ice in a high-speed blender and blend. Pour into a cup and enjoy!

Serves 1

- **½ medium banana (fresh or frozen)**
- **1 big handful spinach**
- **½ cup frozen blueberries**
- **1 scoop (about ⅓ cup) chocolate or vanilla protein powder (at least 20g protein)**
- **1 tablespoon salted, unsweetened peanut butter or almond butter**
- **1 serving of a superfood greens blend (optional)**
- **¾ cup unsweetened almond milk**
- **1 handful ice cubes**

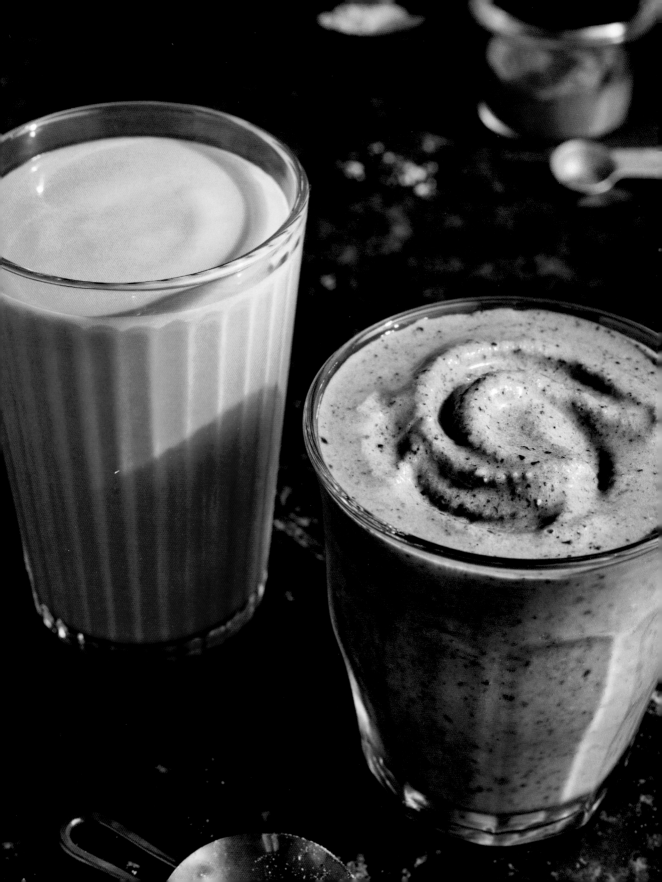

Brain-Boosting Blueberry Milkshake

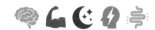

This simple smoothie is excellent for your main brain (in your head) and your second brain (in your belly). The human gut is home to the enteric nervous system, often referred to as the "second brain," which is one of the most influential controllers of our mood, energy, and overall well-being. A healthy gut is a happy gut. Adding in a smoothie like this a couple of times a week is a smart way to support your vitality.

Combine the chia seed gel, almond milk, blueberries, banana, protein powder, yogurt, MCT oil, and ice in a high-speed blender and blend. Pour into a cup and enjoy!

Note: It's a great idea to keep some hydrated chia gel handy for recipes. You can keep a jar of equal parts chia seeds and water (or whatever ratio you prefer), mixed together, in the fridge so you can add chia gel to smoothies whenever you like.

Serves 1

- **2 tablespoon chia seed gel (see Note)**
- **¾ cup unsweetened almond milk**
- **¾ cup frozen blueberries**
- **½ medium banana, peeled, cut in chunks, and frozen**
- **1 scoop (about ⅓ cup) vanilla protein powder (at least 20g protein)**
- **2 tablespoons plain full-fat Greek yogurt**
- **1 tablespoon MCT oil**
- **1 handful ice cubes**

Longevity Shake

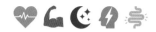

This drink is very special to me. It's my go-to recommendation when someone wants to accelerate their recovery from an injury or they're in need of some deep rejuvenation. One of the highlighted ingredients has been utilized for thousands of years and today, peer-reviewed evidence is revealing why it's so healing and protective. Research cited in the *International Journal of Molecular and Cellular Medicine* found that aloe vera accelerates the healing of tissues, it's anti-inflammatory, blood sugar normalizing, immune system supportive, and even incredibly beneficial for the gut itself. Another ingredient that can be added is colostrum (also known as the "first milk"), which has a variety of rare growth factors and immunomodulating nutrients. When you want to recover, renew, and re-energize your body, this shake has the ingredients to support you.[3]

Combine the blueberries, goji berries, protein powder, aloe vera, colostrum (if using), cashew butter, lion's mane (if using), honey, and ice in a high-speed blender and blend. Pour into a cup and enjoy!

Serves 1

1 cup frozen blueberries

2 tablespoons dried goji berries

1 scoop (about ⅓ cup) chocolate or vanilla protein powder (at least 20g protein; chocolate is ideal)

2 by 2-inch piece fresh aloe vera leaf, filleted from the skin

1 heaping tablespoon colostrum powder (optional)

1 tablespoon cashew butter or 2 tablespoons raw cashews

½ teaspoon lion's mane or other medicinal mushroom (optional)

1 teaspoon raw honey or a few drops of flavored stevia

Pinch of fine sea salt

¾ cup unsweetened almond milk

1 handful ice cubes

Electrolyte Booster

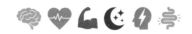

Water and electrolytes are foundational for energy production in our bodies. As we covered earlier, data published in the *International Journal of Environmental Research and Public Health* found that even being mildly dehydrated negatively affects our energy levels, mood, reading speed, and mental work capacity. And by getting properly hydrated, you can rapidly improve all of these things. The truth is, we don't need a fancy nootropic to improve our cognitive performance, we just need water and electrolytes first and foremost! This electrolyte booster utilizes minerals and trace minerals from the citrus, salt, and honey. But you can change it up by going with lemon or lime and utilizing some liquid stevia to keep it truly low-glycemic. I'll have my favorite grab-and-go electrolyte blend that you can keep in your book bag, purse, or travel bag for you in the bonus resources guide at eatsmartercookbook.com/bonus

Combine the water, juice, honey, and salt in a jar with a tight-fitting lid and shake to combine.

Makes about 2½ cups

- **2 cups filtered water or spring water**
- **⅓ cup grapefruit juice (from 1 medium grapefruit)**
- **1 tablespoon raw honey**
- **¼ teaspoon Himalayan salt, Celtic salt, or other high-quality salt**

B's Hot Cocoa

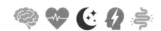

Whenever my youngest son has a day home from school, he loves for me to whip up this superfood hot cocoa as I'm making coffee for my wife and myself. Not only does it provide powerhouse nutrition for his brain and growing body, but it also brings us together for a family ritual in the morning that helps us all connect. Kids and adults alike have thrived utilizing medicinal mushrooms like reishi for thousands of years. One of its most remarkable benefits was highlighted in the journal *Mediators of Inflammation* detailing reishi's elite immune system supportive and anti-inflammatory properties. There are also numerous studies on reishi's ability to help calm the nervous system and even improve sleep quality at night. For instance, a study published in the journal *Pharmacology, Biochemistry, and Behavior* found that reishi has the potential to decrease sleep latency (meaning it helps you fall asleep faster) and was also found to improve the quality of deep sleep. Morning calm and focus, or evening relaxation and recovery—this is a great drink to support your mission.[4,5]

Heat the almond milk in a small saucepan over medium heat until just simmering. Transfer to a blender along with the cacao, collagen peptides, reishi, cinnamon, cardamom, sugar, and stevia. Blend until frothy. Pour into a mug and enjoy!

Note: There's also a great pre-made reishi hot cocoa mixture that we use all the time. I'll have it for you in the bonus resource guide!

Serves 1

- **1 cup unsweetened almond milk**
- **1 tablespoon raw cacao or cocoa powder**
- **1 tablespoon collagen peptides**
- **½ teaspoon reishi or other medicinal mushroom powder**
- **Pinch of ground cinnamon**
- **Pinch of ground cardamom**
- **1 tablespoon coconut sugar or raw honey**
- **A few drops of stevia, or to taste**

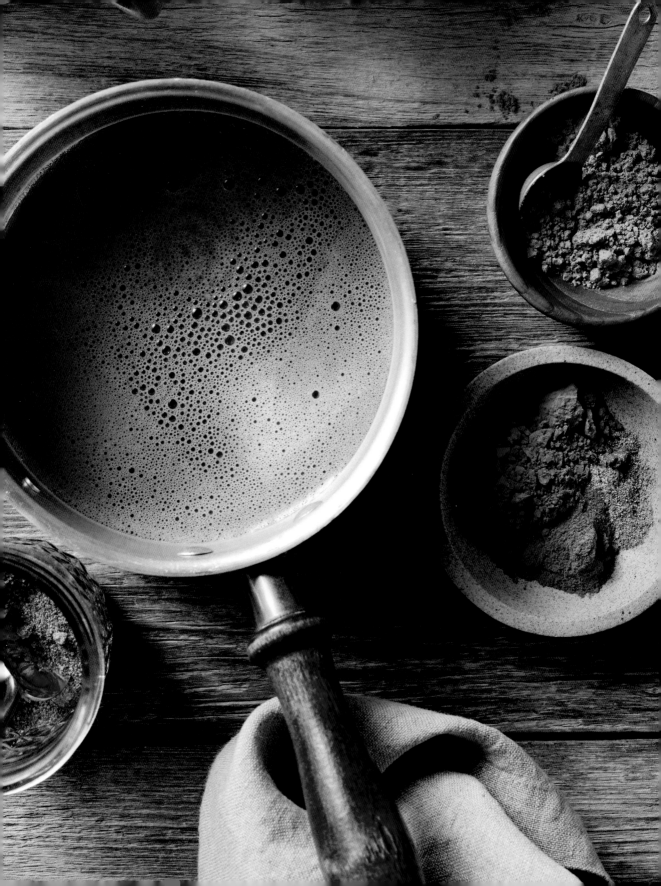

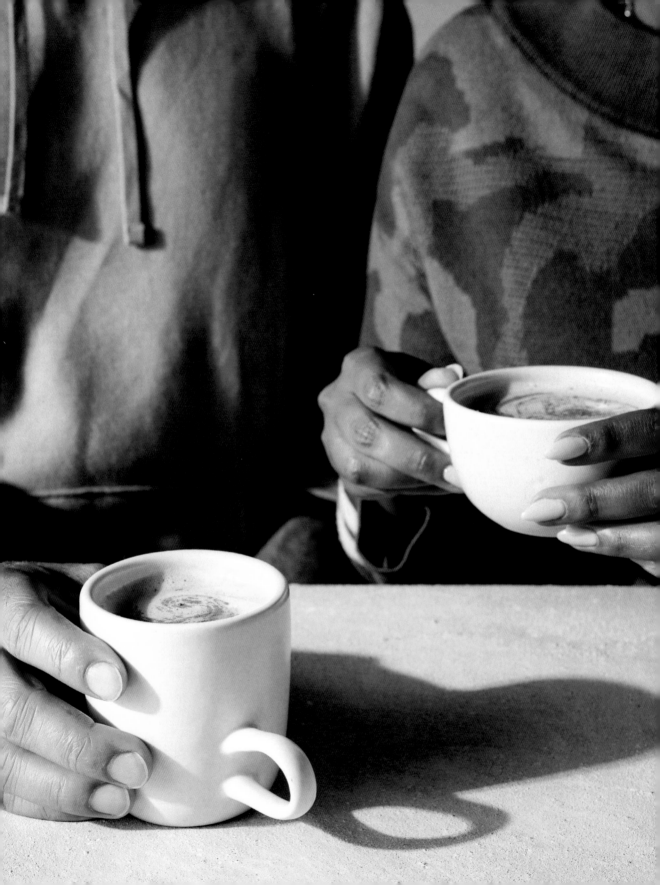

Chai with Ghee

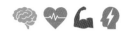

This time-tested combination of tea and spices is delicious and deeply nourishing for your brain and body. The other recipes in this chapter serve one, but because it takes a little time to brew the chai, I decided to make this for two. So if you're only making chai for one, just save the leftover mixture in the fridge so it's ready to reheat and blend with the ghee whenever you're craving some chai! This can easily be scaled up if you want to have some for every day of the week. Feel free to up the black pepper and/or grate in some fresh ginger right before blending if you like it a little spicier!

Combine the water, milk, ginger, cinnamon, cardamom, peppercorns, and honey in a saucepan and bring up to a boil. Partially cover the pan and simmer for 5 minutes to let the flavors infuse.

Turn off the heat, add the tea bags, cover, and let steep for 10 minutes.

Remove the tea bags and strain the liquid into a blender. Add the ghee and blend until emulsified and frothy.

Transfer to small mugs and top each with a pinch of cinnamon.

Serves 2

- **1¼ cups filtered water**
- **1¼ cups unsweetened almond milk or other milk of your choice**
- **1-inch piece fresh ginger, thinly sliced**
- **¼ teaspoon ground cinnamon, plus extra for garnish**
- **⅛ teaspoon ground cardamom**
- **8 black peppercorns**
- **1½ tablespoons raw honey**
- **2 black tea bags (such as English Breakfast) or rooibos if you want something caffeine-free**
- **2 tablespoons grass-fed ghee**

Heart Health Smoothie

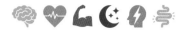

The heavenly chocolate-cherry taste, plus the wide spectrum of supportive nutrients, puts this smoothie in a league of its own! These ingredients are clinically proven to support heart health and defend your cardiovascular system from the leading cause of mortality in our world today. Show your heart some love by enjoying this amazing smoothie a couple of times each week.

Combine the cherries, avocado, cacao powder, hemp seeds, protein powder, almond milk, salt, honey, and ice in a high-speed blender and blend. Pour into a cup, grab a couple of straws if you have some, and enjoy!

Serves 2

2 cups frozen pitted cherries

½ ripe avocado, pitted and peeled

2 teaspoons raw cacao or cocoa powder

¼ cup hulled hemp seeds

2 scoops (about ⅔ cup) chocolate protein powder (at least 20g protein per serving)

1½ cups unsweetened almond milk

Pinch of fine sea salt

1 teaspoon raw honey

2 handfuls ice cubes

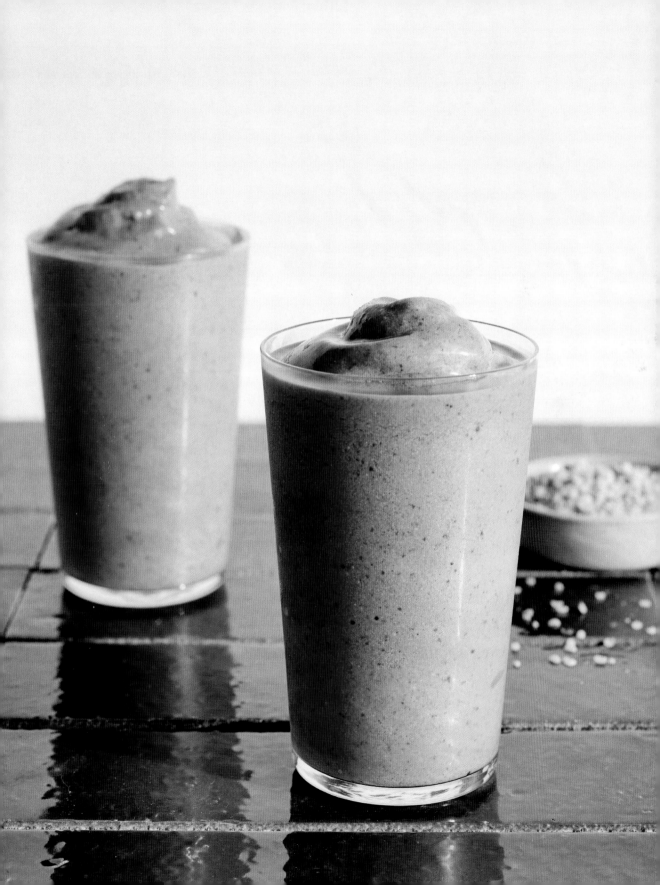

Spa Water

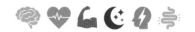

When it comes to hydration, it starts from the top down...literally. According to the journal *Neurology*, even short-term dehydration alarmingly reduces our brain volume—and, thankfully, rehydration rapidly restores it. Here's a refreshing, revitalizing twist to help charge your water up a bit. Proper hydration makes everything in your body work better, and it helps to relax numerous systems in the body, just like a luxurious internal spa day.[6]

Combine the water, cucumber, strawberries, and lemon in a large jug, jar, or pitcher. Cover and place in the fridge for at least 1 hour to infuse. Pour into glasses to serve or if you'd like to remove the fruit garnish, pour through a mesh filter before serving.

Makes about 6 cups

5 cups filtered water

½ cup sliced cucumber

1 cup halved fresh strawberries

1 small organic lemon, thinly sliced

Sweet Potato Pie Smoothie

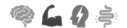

The last place I ever thought I'd see a sweet potato was in a smoothie. But this recipe is undeniably delicious. It's creamy, satisfying, and packed with brain- and metabolism-supportive nutrients. I used a baked sweet potato in this recipe. (I usually bake a few extra and grab them out of the fridge when I'm ready to use them.) But you could also steam, boil, or even use canned sweet potato if you like.

Combine the sweet potato, honey, salt, cinnamon, ginger, cardamom, MCT oil, protein powder, almond milk, and ice in a high-speed blender and blend. Pour into a cup and enjoy!

Serves 1

1 cup cooked sweet potato flesh (from 1 medium/ large sweet potato)

½ teaspoon honey

Pinch of fine sea salt

⅛ teaspoon ground cinnamon

⅛ teaspoon ground ginger

Pinch of ground cardamom

1 tablespoon MCT oil

1 scoop (about ⅓ cup) vanilla protein powder (about 20g protein)

¾ cup unsweetened almond milk (vanilla, if possible)

1 handful ice cubes

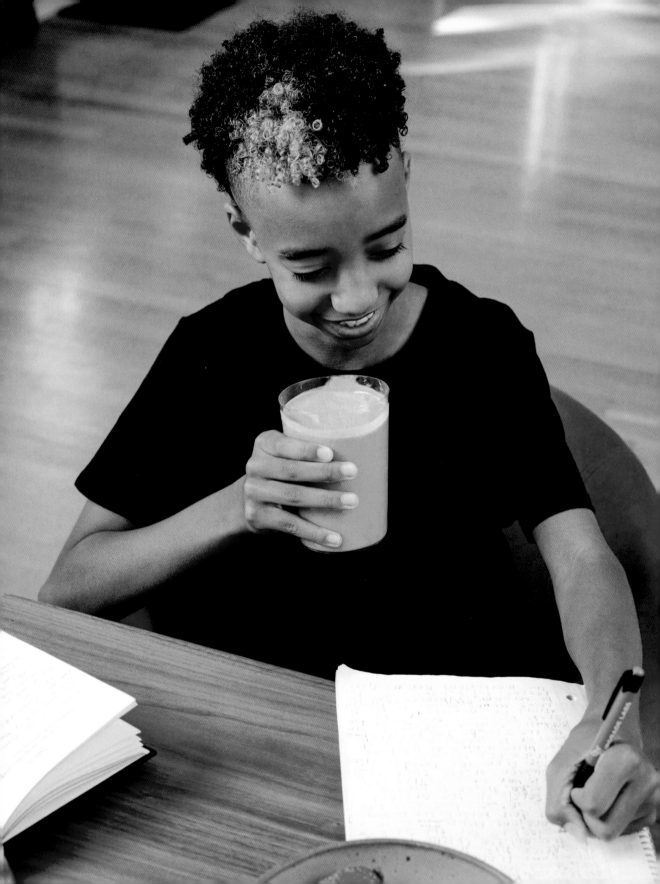

PB&J Superfood Shake

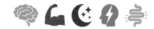

This is an incredible post-workout shake and a family favorite. It has a classic peanut butter and jelly vibe, plus some additional nutrient powerhouses like goji berries to take your recovery up a notch. I'm usually doubling or tripling the recipe when I make it because someone else in my family always wants in on the action.

Mix the chia seeds and water in a small bowl. Stir to combine and let sit for 5 minutes to form a gel.

Add the chia gel to a high-speed blender along with the strawberries, banana, goji berries, protein powder, nut butter, honey, salt, and almond milk and blend. Pour into a cup and enjoy!

Serves 1

1 teaspoon chia seeds

2 to 4 teaspoons water

1¼ cups frozen strawberries

½ cup frozen banana chunks (about ½ banana)

1 tablespoon dried goji berries

1 scoop (about ⅓ cup) vanilla protein powder (at least 20g protein)

1 tablespoon salted, unsweetened peanut butter or almond butter

½ teaspoon raw honey or a few drops of flavored stevia

Small pinch of fine sea salt

¾ cup unsweetened almond milk

Soups & Salads

CHAPTER SIX I'm a huge fan of making a salad into a satisfying, metabolism-supportive meal. These salads, soups, and our family-favorite chili, are guaranteed to give you the deep nutrition and flavor you're looking for!

Smarter Cobb Salad

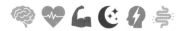

Almost always, restaurants use low-quality vegetable oils for salad dressings. So I wanted to find a way to take advantage of the awesome whole food proteins a Cobb salad delivers, but upgrade the dressing to make it nutrient-dense and delicious. The Smarter Cobb Salad is the ravishing result!

Drizzle the avocado oil in a skillet and add the chicken. Season lightly with salt and pepper. Sauté over medium heat until cooked through and no longer pink, 8 to 10 minutes. Remove from the pan and allow to cool.

Meanwhile, combine the romaine and spinach in a large serving bowl and toss with ¼ cup of the dressing.

Arrange the cooked chicken, sliced eggs, bacon, avocado, blue cheese, and tomatoes on top of the greens. If you'd like more dressing, you can drizzle a little extra over the top. Enjoy!

Serves 4

2 tablespoons avocado oil

4 to 5 boneless skinless chicken thighs (about 1½ pounds total), chopped

Sea salt and black pepper

3 cups chopped romaine lettuce (1 small romaine heart)

3 cups baby spinach firmly packed, roughly chopped if large

3 hard-boiled large organic eggs, peeled and sliced

6 slices bacon, cooked and crumbled

1 ripe medium avocado, pitted, peeled, and sliced or diced

⅓ cup crumbled blue cheese or other grated cheese of your choice

2 medium tomatoes, diced

Honey Mustard Dressing (page 280)

Prebiotic-Boosting Spinach Salad

This simple, tasty salad provides an array of prebiotic plant fibers that support the health of your microbiome. Most notably, the artichokes, olives, and onions are all shown in peer-reviewed data to aid in probiotic diversity, reduce inflammation, and improve metabolic health. This is an awesome side salad or appetizer. To make it a meal, just add your protein of choice![7]

Place spinach in a serving bowl and top with the olives, onion, and feta. Sprinkle over the Italian seasoning and vinaigrette, and toss to combine. Season to taste with salt and pepper, if desired.

Serves 4

5 (5-ounce) containers baby spinach

1 cup chopped drained marinated artichoke hearts

½ cup chopped pitted kalamata olives

¼ small red onion, thinly sliced

½ cup crumbled feta cheese

1 teaspoon Italian seasoning

3 tablespoons Simple and Smart Vinaigrette (page 278)

Sea salt and black pepper

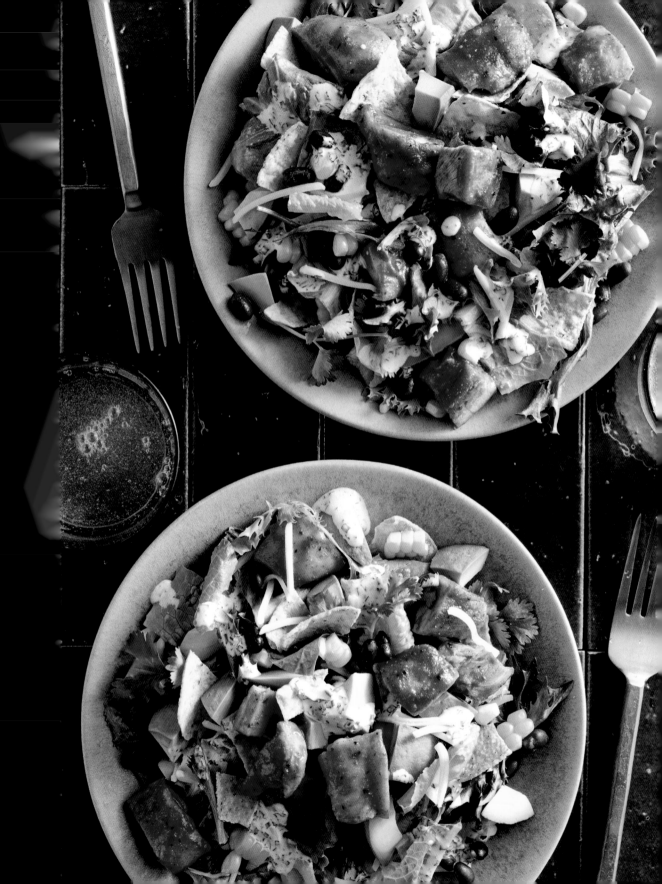

Southwest BBQ Chicken Salad

The variety of flavors and nutrients come together to make this salad truly special. It's my youngest son's favorite...so it's definitely kid tested and *Eat Smarter* approved!

Preheat the oven to 375°F.

Season the chicken thighs with the salt, pepper, onion powder, garlic powder, and paprika and arrange them on a baking sheet. Transfer to the oven and bake for 30 to 35 minutes, until cooked through.

Take out the chicken and cut it into dice. Return the chicken to the baking sheet and pour over the barbecue sauce, making sure it's evenly distributed. Reduce the oven temperature to 250°F and place the chicken back in the oven for another 10 to 15 minutes, until nicely glazed.

Combine the spring mix, romaine, corn, black beans, cheese, and cilantro in a large serving bowl. Toss with the ranch dressing, check for seasoning, and add more salt and/or pepper if necessary.

Top the salad with the cooked chicken, tortilla chips, and avocado, if using.

Serves 4

- **6 boneless skinless chicken thighs (about 2 pounds total)**
- **½ teaspoon kosher salt**
- **½ teaspoon black pepper**
- **1 teaspoon onion powder**
- **1 teaspoon garlic powder**
- **1 teaspoon paprika**
- **1½ cups barbecue sauce (365 Organic Memphis Madness sauce is our go-to)**
- **3 cups spring greens mix firmly packed, chopped**
- **3 cups chopped romaine lettuce (1 small romaine heart)**
- **1 cup yellow corn kernels (heated and drained if frozen)**
- **1 cup black beans (rinsed and drained canned or home-cooked)**
- **¾ cup shredded cheese (your choice; about 3 ounces)**
- **1 handful fresh cilantro leaves, roughly chopped**
- **¾ cup Smarter Ranch Dressing (page 286)**
- **1 cup crushed tortilla chips**
- **1½ avocados, pitted, peeled, and diced (optional)**

Superfood Salad

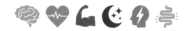

What happens when your salad gets endowed with superpowers? You get this! The powerful combination of whole foods, superfoods, and flavor just might ignite your superhuman abilities, too. This salad is packed with plant-based proteins. You can easily omit the chicken and make it a satisfying vegetarian version. Also, I like to spice things up from time to time (literally), so I'll add a few pinches of cayenne pepper!

In a large salad bowl, combine the greens with the vinaigrette and spirulina and toss to coat. Divide between four bowls or serve family style on a large platter. Top with the avocado, chicken, tomato, hemp seeds, and pumpkin seeds (if using), and give it a light toss.

Grab a fork and enjoy!

Serves 4

6 cups torn spinach, romaine lettuce, and/or mixed salad greens

½ cup Simple and Smart Vinaigrette (page 278)

2 teaspoons spirulina powder

1 ripe avocado, peeled, pitted, and chopped

2 or 3 grilled chicken breasts (about 1 pound), chopped or diced (see Note)

2 medium tomatoes, diced, or 1½ cups cherry tomatoes, halved

¼ cup hulled hemp seeds

½ cup sprouted pumpkin seeds or sunflower seeds (if you want a little extra crunch; optional)

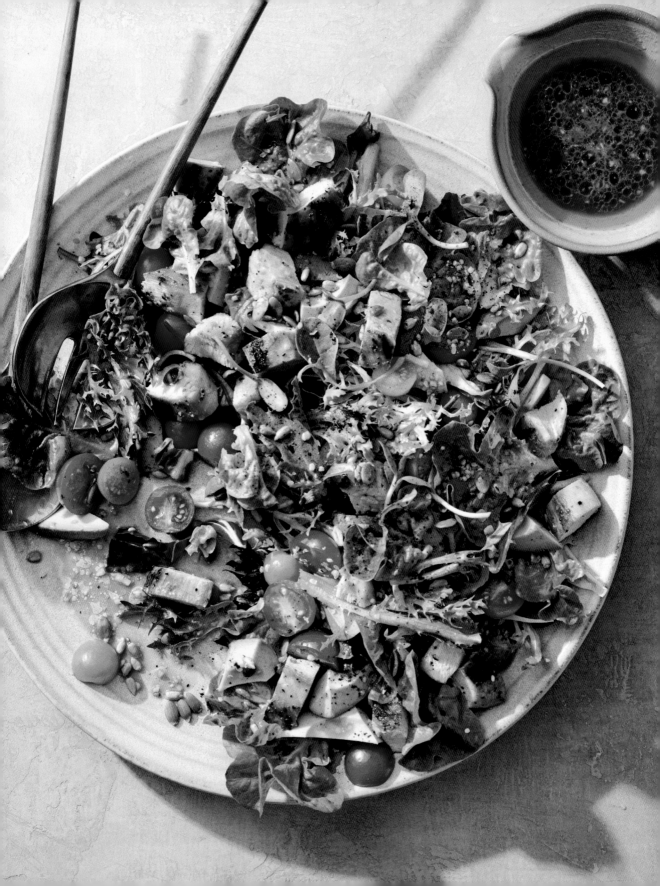

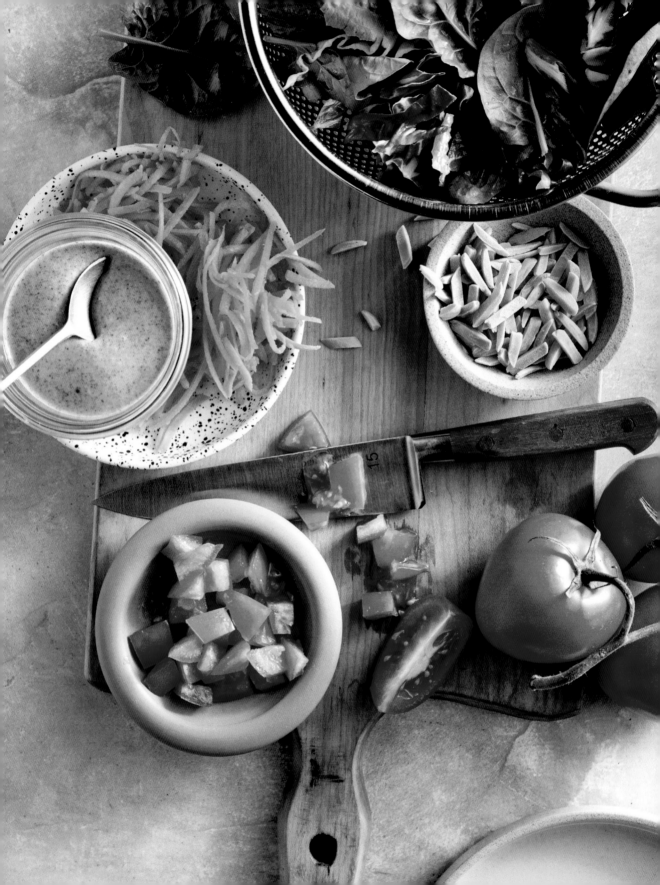

Gratitude Salad

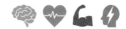

This amazing salad features the very first homemade dressing I ever had. My mom-in-law made it for me at a time when eating a salad was brand-new in my life. Believe it or not, coming from my heavily processed–food upbringing, I didn't have my first salad until I was 25 years old! This salad, and this incredible dressing, bridged the gap. I couldn't believe that a salad could taste so flavorful and fulfilling. Since my wife and mom-in-law are from Kenya, I named the dressing Asante Sana, which means "thank you very much" in Swahili.

This is a wonderful side salad, but you can easily include some additional protein (steak or fish would be great) to make it a full-on meal.

Combine the lettuce, tomatoes, carrot, and avocado in a large bowl. Toss with the dressing and season to taste with salt and pepper. Sprinkle over the almonds and serve.

Serves 4 to 6

5 (5-ounce) containers mixed greens or 6 cups chopped romaine lettuce

½ cup chopped tomatoes

1 large carrot, grated

½ cup Asante Sana Dressing (page 283)

Sea salt and black pepper

⅓ cup toasted slivered almonds

Lentil Salad with Broccoli and Spinach

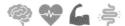

I love salads that are versatile, meaning that they can be eaten as a side or as a satisfying meal on their own. This nutrient-rich salad works great paired with a simply cooked protein for dinner, and can also make a hearty lunch all by itself. You can easily make a batch of it, store it in some smart containers (as we covered in Chapter Two) and have it for lunch for a couple of days. The feta adds nice salt and tang, but feel free to leave it out to make this a totally vegan dish if that suits your fancy.

Bring a large pot of water up to a boil. Add the broccoli and cook for about 2 to 3 minutes, until bright green but not soft. Drain, rinse under cold water to cool down fast, then drain well and chop.

Combine the broccoli, lentils, spinach, onion, feta, and walnuts in a large bowl. Toss with the dressing and season to taste with salt and pepper.

Serves 4

2 cups chopped broccoli florets (roughly 1-inch pieces)

2 cups cooked lentils, drained

1 cup packed baby spinach, roughly chopped

¼ cup minced red onion

⅓ cup crumbled feta cheese (optional)

⅓ cup chopped toasted walnuts

3 tablespoons Honey Mustard Dressing (page 280), or to taste

Sea salt and black pepper

Protein-Packed Sardine Salad

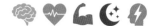

I remember my mom eating sardines when I was a kid, and I thought it was one of the freakiest things I'd ever seen. It took years before I put my fishy bias to the side and looked into the nutrition and history of sardines. Humans have been preserving fish for thousands of years. Sardines rose to the top in popularity thanks in large part to their omega-3 fatty acid and abundance of micronutrients. Just 3½ ounces of sardines provides more than 150 percent of the RDA for vitamin B$_{12}$ and 63 percent of the RDA for vitamin D. This salad is a wonderful combination of nutrient-dense foods and flavors that will wow your taste buds.

Bring a pot of water up to a boil and add some kosher salt. Cook the potatoes in the boiling water until very tender, about 15 minutes. Drain and set aside to cool a bit.

Meanwhile, for the dressing, whisk together the vinegar, mustard, shallot, and olive oil and season to taste with sea salt and pepper.

Cut the potatoes into ½-inch slices and toss in a serving bowl with the dressing. Add the olives, capers, eggs, and sardines and toss to combine. Mix in the arugula and serve.

Note: The quality of this dish really depends on the quality of sardines you use, so be sure to purchase them packed in extra virgin olive oil or water, and avoid sardines packed in lower-quality oils.

Serves 4

- ¾ pound fingerling or small Yukon gold potatoes, peeled if you prefer
- 2 tablespoons red wine vinegar
- 1 teaspoon Dijon mustard
- 1 small/medium shallot, thinly sliced
- ¼ cup olive oil
- Sea salt and black pepper
- ¼ cup pitted kalamata or similar olives, roughly chopped
- 2 tablespoons capers, drained and rinsed (optional)
- 4 hard-boiled large organic eggs, peeled and quartered
- 1 (3- to 4-ounce) can good-quality sardines in olive oil, drained and cut or broken into small pieces (see Note)
- 4 handfuls baby arugula

Cucumber Salad

This simple, refreshing salad is my wife's favorite. The recipe is a collaborative effort of her sister, Mukami (who's another amazing cook), and my mom-in-law. It's packed with micronutrients and phenomenal for keeping everything moving in the right direction with your digestive health. It's an awesome side salad to have anytime you want to upgrade the nutrient density of any meal.

Slice the cucumbers in half lengthwise, then roughly chop. Transfer to a large bowl. Mix in the bell pepper, tomato, and onion. Add the olive oil, vinegar, and dulse flakes (if using), and season with salt and pepper to taste.

Toss to combine and add more oil, vinegar, salt, and/or pepper to taste. Serve immediately. Or if you have time, cover with plastic wrap and refrigerate for an hour to let the veggies marinate.

Serves 2 to 4

5 or 6 Persian cucumbers or 1 large English cucumber

½ red bell pepper, seeded and diced

½ roma tomato, seeded and diced

¼ red or white onion, thinly sliced

1 tablespoon olive oil

2 to 3 tablespoons white or apple cider vinegar

½ teaspoon dulse flakes (optional)

Sea salt and black pepper

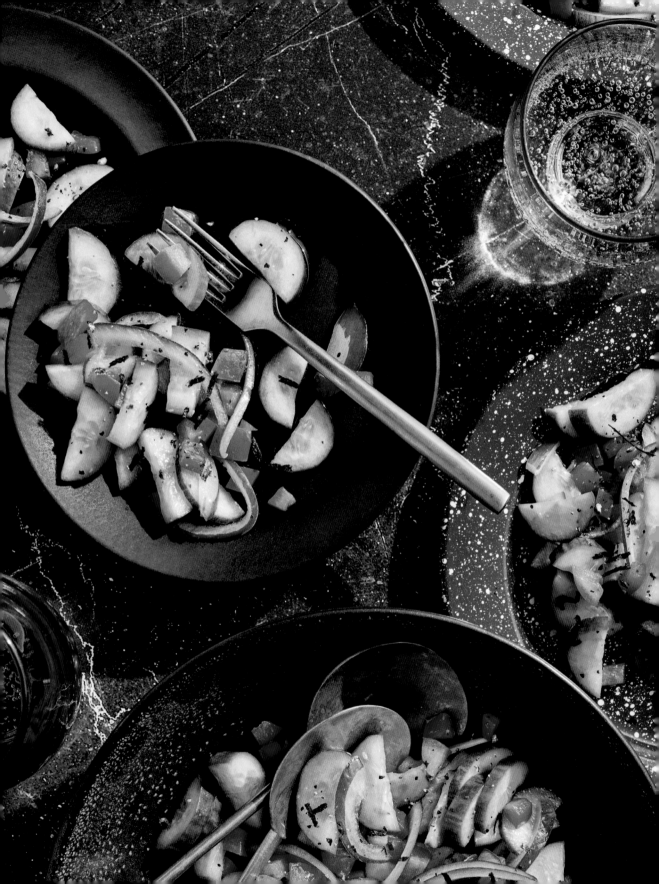

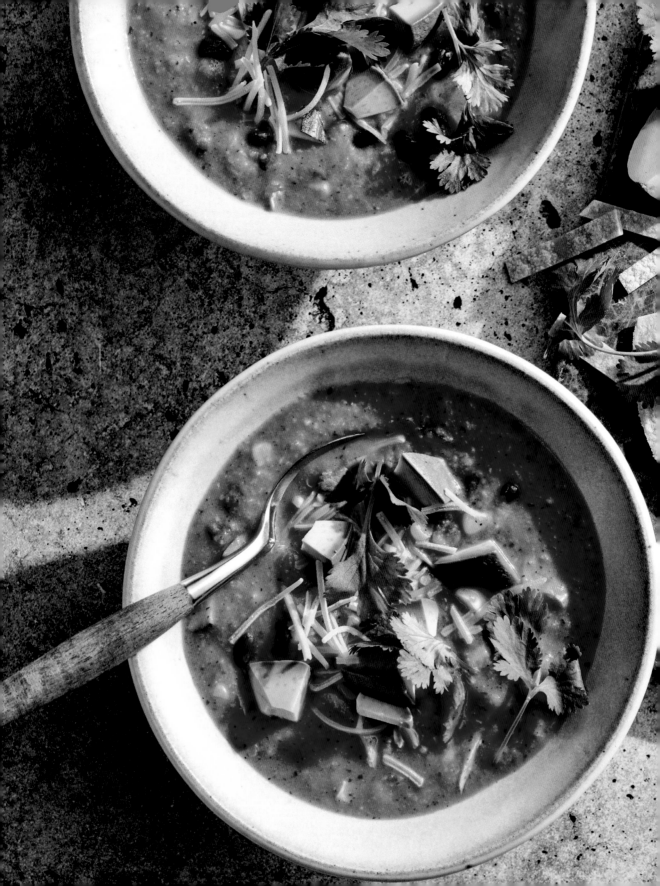

Tortilla Soup

This soup is next level! Growing up, my only trysts with soup were canned chicken noodle or tomato soups. I had no idea that soups could be so fresh, so fulfilling, and so delicious. This wonderful recipe combines a variety of metabolism- *and* microbiome-supportive ingredients into one flavorful dish.

Heat the avocado oil in a medium Dutch oven over medium heat. Add the onion and bell pepper, season generously with salt and pepper, and sauté for 5 minutes, until the onion is translucent and starting to brown.

Add the garlic, cumin, ground chipotle, cilantro, and tortilla strips. Sauté for another 2 minutes, stirring to make sure nothing sticks to the bottom. (You can add a splash more oil if things are getting too dry or starting to burn.)

Add the tomatoes, rinse out the can with the water, and pour that in, too. Turn the heat down to low and simmer for 5 minutes.

Add the chicken broth and bring it up to a boil. Partially cover, reduce the heat to maintain a simmer, and cook for 20 minutes.

Turn off the heat and carefully blend the soup in the pot with an immersion blender. Add the zucchini, corn, and beans. Turn the heat back on to low and simmer for 5 minutes or until the zucchini is just cooked through. Taste for seasoning and add more salt and pepper if desired.

Serve with cheese, avocado, and more cilantro on top!

Note: You can sub in store-bought rotisserie chicken for the cooked chicken breast if you ever want to save a few minutes. Rotisserie chickens are generally not very expensive and can be used to make a variety of dishes, so it's nice to have one handy.

Serves 4 to 6

- **2 tablespoons avocado oil, plus extra if needed**
- **1 medium yellow onion, diced**
- **½ red bell pepper, seeded and diced**
- **Sea salt and black pepper**
- **2 garlic cloves, minced**
- **½ teaspoon ground cumin**
- **¼ teaspoon ground chipotle**
- **¼ cup chopped fresh cilantro leaves, plus extra leaves for serving**
- **2 corn tortillas, cut into ¼-inch-wide strips**
- **1 (15-ounce) can fire-roasted diced tomatoes (don't drain!)**
- **¼ cup water**
- **3 cups chicken or veggie broth**
- **1 medium zucchini, diced (about 1½ cups)**
- **½ cup frozen corn kernels**
- **½ cup drained cooked black beans**
- **1 cooked chicken breast, boned, skinned, and shredded (optional; see Note)**
- **Grated cheese (such as Monterey Jack)**
- **Diced ripe avocado**

Slow Cooker Beef Chili

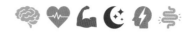

Few things are as heart-warming as a bowl of chili made by someone you love. This chili is power-packed with veggies. Plus, it features a special star ingredient (cacao!) that's going to bring everything together and knock your socks off. The ingredient list looks long, but it's fairly simple to throw together, makes a big batch, and freezes well!

Heat a large Dutch oven over medium heat. Add the avocado oil, onion, and bell pepper and sauté for 5 minutes or until the onion is translucent and starting to brown. Add the mushrooms and garlic and cook for another 5 minutes. Transfer the veggies to the slow cooker (see Note).

Add the ground beef to the Dutch oven. Sauté over medium-high heat for about 5 minutes, using a spatula or wooden spoon to break up the meat into small pieces. When the meat has browned, add the cumin, onion powder, garlic powder, ground chipotle, paprika, and cinnamon and cook for another minute. Add the broth to the pan and use the spatula to scrape up any browned bits stuck to the bottom. Carefully transfer the beef mixture to the slow cooker.

Stir in the beans, tomatoes, sweet potato, cacao, sugar, vinegar, and salt. Set the slow cooker to low, cover, and cook for 6 hours.

Stir in the spinach and let it wilt for 5 minutes.

Divide the chili between serving bowls and let people choose their favorite garnishes.

Serves 6 to 8

3 tablespoons avocado oil

1 large yellow onion, finely diced

½ red bell pepper, seeded and finely diced

½ pound cremini mushrooms, finely diced

4 garlic cloves, minced

1 pound 80/20 ground grass-fed beef

1 teaspoon ground cumin

1 teaspoon onion powder

1 teaspoon garlic powder

½ teaspoon ground chipotle

2 teaspoons smoked paprika

¼ teaspoon ground cinnamon

1 cup Beef Bone Broth (page 170) or water

1 (15-ounce) can black beans, rinsed and drained

1 (15-ounce) can pinto beans, rinsed and drained

1 (15-ounce) can diced fire-roasted tomatoes (don't drain!)

1 medium sweet potato, peeled and cut into ½-inch pieces

1 teaspoon raw cacao or cocoa powder

2 teaspoons coconut sugar

1½ tablespoons apple cider vinegar

1½ teaspoons kosher salt

3 cups baby spinach firmly packed, roughly chopped

Garnishes such as grated cheese, sour cream, hot sauce, pickled jalapeños, and fresh cilantro

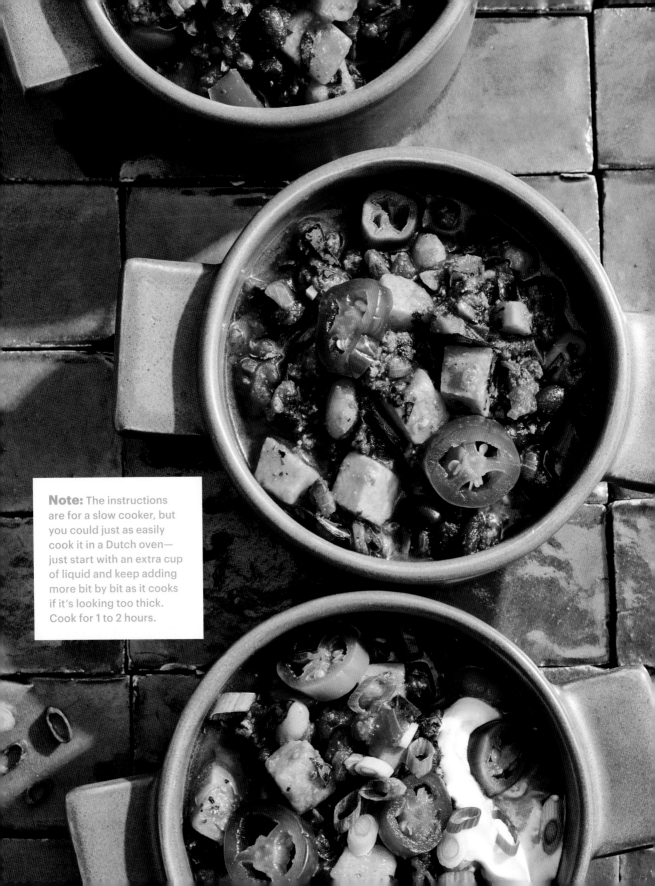

Note: The instructions are for a slow cooker, but you could just as easily cook it in a Dutch oven— just start with an extra cup of liquid and keep adding more bit by bit as it cooks if it's looking too thick. Cook for 1 to 2 hours.

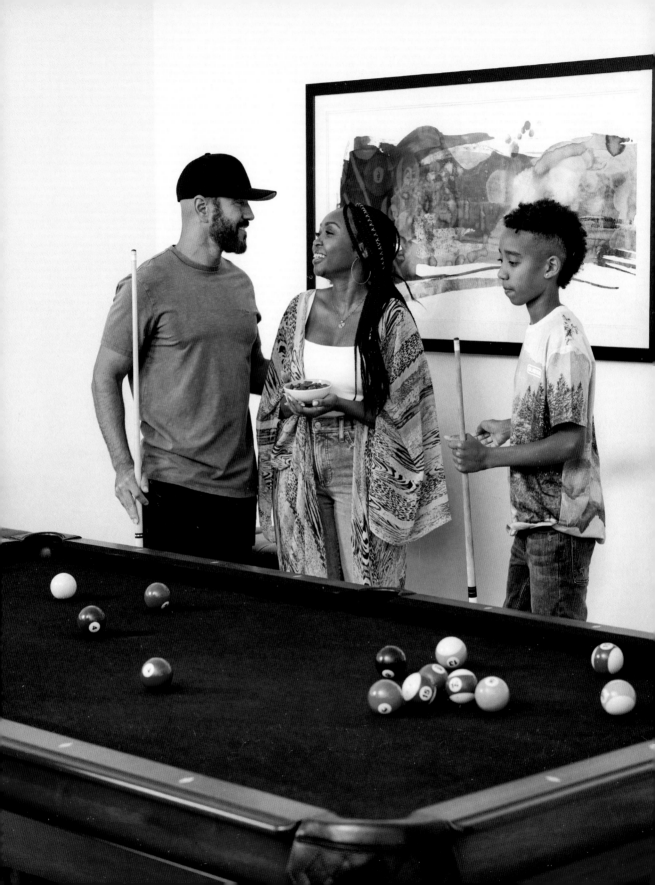

Beef Bone Broth

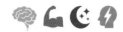

Bone broth has been a staple in human culture for thousands of years. The abundance of micronutrients found in bone broth is truly unique. Combine that with the rich amount of the amino acid glycine, and it's excellent for your skin, bone health, joint health, and more. A study cited in the journal *Current Opinion in Clinical Nutrition and Metabolic Care* detailed the remarkable anti-inflammatory and immune system–supportive benefits that glycine has. You can generally find bones to use for broth at your local grocery store's meat department. Ideally, get grass-fed bones whenever possible. This recipe is really the base model. I highly recommend adding additional fresh herbs and spices you enjoy, like bay leaves, oregano, or cilantro, just to name a few.[8]

Preheat the oven to 350°F.

Place the beef bones on a baking sheet and roast for 30 minutes or until browned.

Transfer the bones to a slow cooker and pour over the water and vinegar. Let sit for 20 to 30 minutes. (The acid helps make the nutrients in the bones more available.)

Roughly chop the onion, carrots, and celery and add to the pot along with the salt and pepper. Turn the slow cooker on low and cook for 48 hours.

Add the garlic powder and paprika, if using, and cook for another 30 minutes.

Turn off the slow cooker and let the broth cool slightly. Strain into a gallon-sized container using a fine-mesh strainer to remove all the bits of bone and vegetable. When cool enough, transfer to a large glass jar or smaller mason jars and store in the fridge for up to 5 days or freeze for later use.

Makes about 4 quarters; serves 2 to 4

- **2 pounds beef bones (from a healthy source, preferably grass-fed)**
- **1 gallon (4 quarts) filtered water**
- **2 tablespoons apple cider vinegar**
- **1 onion**
- **2 carrots**
- **3 celery stalks**
- **1 tablespoon kosher salt**
- **1 teaspoon black pepper**
- **1 tablespoon garlic powder (optional)**
- **1 tablespoon paprika (optional)**

Bowls, Burgers & Wraps

CHAPTER SEVEN   One of the most amazing things about building real-food bowls is the endless combinations. Diversity is a hallmark of microbial health. A recent study published in the *International Journal of Obesity* revealed that a higher diversity of gut bacteria is directly correlated with less weight gain and improved energy metabolism *independent of calorie intake and other factors*. The number one way to increase the diversity of your microbiome is to increase the variety of foods that you're eating. These mouthwatering bowls, burgers, and wraps are a family-friendly way to help get you there.[9]

Harvest Bowl with Honey Mustard

This bowl fueled my mind and body while writing this cookbook on more than one occasion. I absolutely love the combination of tastes and textures. The spicy mixed nuts take this bowl to another level, but toasted walnuts, pistachios, or slivered almonds can work great, too.

Preheat the oven to 400°F. Line a baking sheet with parchment paper.

Toss the sweet potato with 1 tablespoon of the olive oil and season with salt and pepper. Toss the chicken thighs with the remaining olive oil and the garlic powder and paprika, and season generously with salt and pepper. Arrange the sweet potato and chicken on the baking sheet and roast in the oven for 35 minutes or until the chicken is cooked through and no longer pink inside.

Remove the chicken to a cutting board and chop it into bite-sized pieces.

To assemble the bowls, place ¾ cup quinoa in each bowl, then top with one-quarter each of the sweet potato, chicken, kale, and nuts. Drizzle over the dressing and enjoy!

Serves 4

1 large sweet potato, scrubbed and cut into ½-inch dice

2 tablespoons olive oil

Sea salt and black pepper

6 boneless skinless chicken thighs (about 1¼ pounds total)

½ teaspoon garlic powder

½ teaspoon paprika

3 cups cooked quinoa

4 small handfuls baby kale

½ cup Smoky Spicy Mixed Nuts (page 247)

½ cup Honey Mustard Dressing (page 280), or to taste

Smarter Burrito Bowl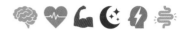

Plenty of places offer burrito bowls today, but making them at home is a fun, tasty way to improve the quality of ingredients that are used—especially the oils that are used in the cooking process. It's easy to make a lower-carb variation of this by swapping the rice for cauliflower rice and omitting the beans.

Heat a grill pan over medium-high heat. Toss the chicken thighs with 1 tablespoon of the oil, the garlic powder, and paprika, and season generously with salt and pepper. Grill for about 5 minutes per side, until cooked through. Remove to a cutting board to rest for at least 5 minutes before dicing.

Heat a large sauté pan over medium-high heat. Add the remaining avocado oil and throw in the onions and peppers. Cook for about 5 minutes, stirring often, until the veggies are tender and starting to char in places.

To assemble the bowls, divide the rice between four serving bowls. Top each one with one-quarter each of the pepper and onion mixture, chicken, salsa, guacamole, cheese and greens. Garnish with add-ins of choice and serve.

Serves 4

6 boneless skinless chicken thighs (about 2 pounds)

3 tablespoons avocado oil

1 teaspoon garlic powder

1 teaspoon paprika

Sea salt and black pepper

½ red or yellow onion, thinly sliced

1 red, yellow, or orange bell pepper, seeded and thinly sliced

2 cups cooked rice (your choice) or cauliflower rice

½ cup pico de gallo or salsa of your choice

½ cup Speedy Superfood Guacamole (page 244) or diced ripe avocado

¾ cup shredded cheese of your choice (about 3 ounces)

1 cup spring greens mix or chopped romaine lettuce

ADD-INS AND GARNISHES IF YOU DESIRE

Drained cooked black or pinto beans (ideally cooked with a pressure cooker)

Sour cream

Crushed tortilla chips

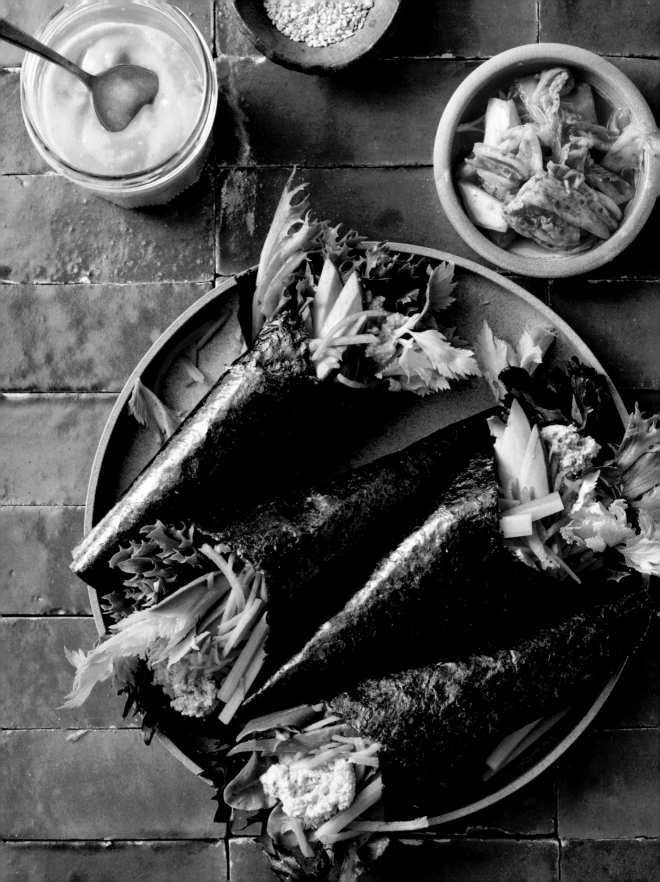

Faux Salmon Nori Wraps

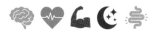

Some dishes are so good (yet unsuspecting) that you have to taste them to believe it! One of the first times we made this dish was during a nutrition/food tasting class my wife and I put together back in 2009. I remember it so clearly, because we left the class and headed straight to the theater to see *Transformers: Revenge of the Fallen*. I can tell you one thing, the walnuts in this recipe transform into a delicious faux salmon pâté far more effortlessly than the *Transformers* franchise trying to transition from Shia LaBeouf to Mark Wahlberg. If you know, then you know! I love serving these sushi rolls with miso mayo for dipping, but I also love them with a simple dipping sauce of soy sauce, rice vinegar, and sesame seeds, too. The wrapping and rolling may take a bit of practice, but even if your wraps aren't picture perfect, they are guaranteed to be delicious. Just be sure to eat them soon after rolling, because the nori starts to soften as it sits.

To make the faux salmon pâté, combine the walnuts, celery, bell pepper, onion, and salt in a food processor and blend until smooth.

To assemble the wraps, take a sheet of nori, spread 1 cup of the spring mix down the center, then top with one-quarter each of the pâté, grated carrot, celery, and avocado. Carefully roll up the wrap (see Note). Repeat with the remaining sheets of nori and fillings. You can slice the rolls into standard sushi bites, or enjoy the sushi roll burrito style. Serve immediately with kimchi on the side and miso mayo for dipping.

Note: It's not necessary to have a sushi rolling mat, but if you have one, it's made for moments like this!

Serves 2 to 4

FAUX SALMON PÂTÉ

- **1 cup walnut halves and pieces, soaked in warm water for 1 hour and drained**
- **1 celery stalk, roughly chopped**
- **½ large red bell pepper, seeded and roughly chopped**
- **2 tablespoons diced red onion**
- **¾ teaspoon kosher salt**

WRAPS

- **4 sheets toasted nori**
- **4 cups spring mix**
- **1 carrot, grated**
- **1 celery stalk, cut into matchsticks**
- **1 ripe avocado, pitted, peeled, and sliced**

TO SERVE

- **1 cup roughly chopped kimchi**
- **Miso Mayo (page 281)**

Pesto Turkey Wrap

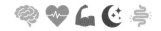

There was a time in my life when I was legitimately wrapped up in making wraps. Some people have a "goth" phase, I had a "wrapping every conceivable combination of foods up in a tortilla or collard leaf" phase. Thankfully, all of the experimentation brought me to a place of knowing what makes a truly elite, real-food wrap. This recipe serves as a great grab-and-go lunch. And for a variation, you can easily sub in grilled chicken instead of turkey.

Place a lavash wrap on a cutting board and spread 1 tablespoon of the mayo and 1 tablespoon of the pesto in the center. Top with ¼ pound of the sliced turkey, then one-quarter each of the avocado, roasted peppers, and mozzarella. Season with a pinch of salt and pepper and arrange one-quarter of the greens on top. Gently roll up into a wrap. Repeat with the remaining 3 lavash and the rest of the fillings and enjoy!

Serves 4

4 lavash wraps or burrito-sized tortillas

¼ cup mayo (avocado oil-based mayo is ideal)

¼ cup Superfood Pesto (page 284) or your favorite store-bought pesto

1 pound sliced nitrate-free roasted turkey breast

1 ripe avocado, pitted, peeled, and sliced

⅓ cup jarred roasted bell peppers, thinly sliced

1 (4-ounce) ball fresh mozzarella cheese in water, sliced

Sea salt and black pepper

1½ cups baby arugula or spinach

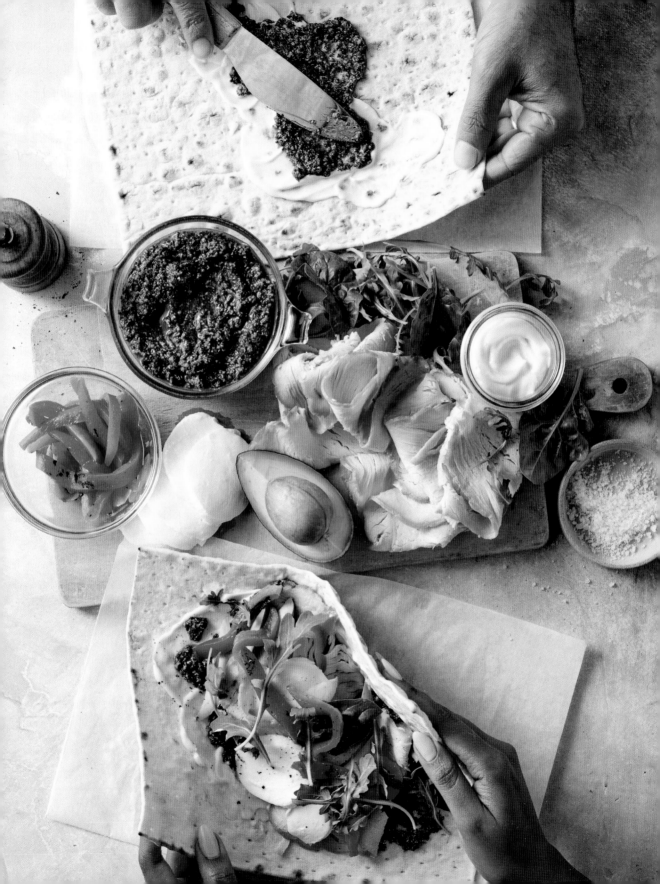

Salmon, Kale, and Kraut Bowl

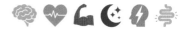

Getting in a few servings of fermented foods each week can be amazing for your gut health and metabolism. A study published in the journal *PLoS One* found that lactobacillus, a probiotic strain found in sauerkraut, can potentially defend against fat gain by modulating genes associated with metabolism and inflammation in the liver and adipose tissue. How is this possible? It's because bacteria aren't just assistants in our digestive health; they also influence our genetic expression! Typically, probiotic-rich sauerkraut will be found in the refrigerated section, but still check the label to be sure. Make sure to avoid purchasing pasteurized off-the-shelf versions of sauerkraut because the vast majority of the probiotics will have been destroyed. Combining kraut with the metabolic- and brain-boosting benefits of the greens and salmon, this bowl is certified to support your health and well-being.[10]

Combine the kale, lemon juice, olive oil, and soy sauce in a medium bowl. Season lightly with salt and pepper. Use your hands to massage the kale until slightly softened. Set aside.

Divide the rice between four bowls. Top each bowl with one-quarter of the salmon, one-quarter of the avocado, ¼ cup of the sauerkraut, and one-quarter of the massaged kale.

Drizzle or spoon 1 tablespoon of the mayo over each bowl and garnish with sesame and hemp seeds. Serve with extra mayo, lemon wedges, and sriracha on the side, if you like.

Serves 4

1 bunch lacinato kale (aka dino kale), ribs removed, thinly sliced

1 tablespoon fresh lemon juice

3 tablespoons olive oil

1 tablespoon soy sauce

Sea salt and black pepper

3 cups cooked brown rice

1 pound Honey Sriracha Salmon (page 193; two 8-ounce fillets) or simply cooked salmon

1 ripe large avocado, pitted, peeled, and sliced or diced

1 cup sauerkraut, drained well

¼ cup Miso Mayo (page 281), plus extra for serving if desired

About 1 tablespoon toasted sesame seeds

About 1 tablespoon hulled hemp seeds

Lemon wedges and sriracha hot sauce (optional)

Greek Quinoa Bowl with Chicken Meatballs

Good meatballs are hard to beat. The mayo in this recipe keeps these meatballs nice and moist. Along with the olives, arugula, and other veggies, the flavor combinations are just amazing. I use an avocado oil–based mayo, but feel free to use your favorite kind (avoiding low-quality oils, of course!). You could also sub in grilled chicken or salmon, or even more veggies and feta for a vegetarian spin. The Italian Dressing on page 287 is perfect here, but if you're in a pinch and don't have time to make it, a drizzle of apple cider vinegar and olive oil works well coming off the bench.

Preheat the oven to 425°F. Lightly grease a baking sheet with the avocado oil.

Combine the ground chicken, salt, Italian seasoning, garlic powder, onion powder, parsley, and mayo in a medium bowl. Mix with your hands gently but thoroughly. Form into 16 walnut-sized meatballs. Arrange on the baking sheet and bake for 15 minutes or until very firm when pressed. Turn on the broiler and cook for another 2 to 5 minutes, until the tops are nicely browned.

Divide the cooked quinoa between four bowls. Top each with a handful of arugula and one-quarter each of the tomatoes, cucumber, feta, and olives. Add 4 meatballs to each bowl and drizzle over a couple of tablespoons of Italian dressing.

Serves 4

MEATBALLS

1 teaspoon avocado oil

1 pound ground dark meat chicken

1 teaspoon kosher salt

1 teaspoon Italian seasoning

½ teaspoon garlic powder

½ teaspoon onion powder

2 tablespoons finely chopped fresh parsley

2 tablespoons of your favorite mayo

BOWLS

3 cups cooked quinoa

4 handfuls baby arugula

1 cup chopped tomatoes

1 cup chopped cucumber

1 cup crumbled feta cheese (about 4 ounces)

½ cup pitted kalamata olives

½ cup Italian Dressing (page 287)

Kimchi Cauliflower Bowl

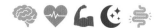

As noted in Chapter Three, kimchi is another time-tested food that has bona fide antiobesity effects. This flavorful bowl is easy to put together and great for breakfast, lunch, or dinner.

Heat a large sauté pan over medium heat. Add 2 tablespoons of the avocado oil and the cauliflower and kale. Season to taste with salt and pepper and cook for 5 to 8 minutes, until the cauliflower is tender and starting to brown. Add the garlic and ginger and sauté for another minute.

In a separate safe nonstick pan, heat the remaining oil over medium-high heat. Crack in the eggs, season with salt and pepper, and cook for 4 to 6 minutes until the whites are set and the yolks are still runny.

Divide the quinoa between four bowls. Top each with one-quarter of the cauliflower and kale mixture, 1 egg, and ¼ cup of the kimchi. Drizzle over 1 tablespoon of the soy sauce and enjoy!

Serves 4

4 tablespoons avocado oil

½ small/medium head cauliflower, finely chopped (about 3 cups)

½ bunch dino kale, stems removed and roughly chopped

Sea salt and black pepper

2 garlic cloves, minced

1-inch piece ginger, peeled and minced

4 large organic eggs

3 cups cooked quinoa

1 cup kimchi, drained and chopped

4 tablespoons soy sauce

Smarter Veggie Burgers

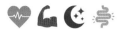

I know what it's like to look for a healthy plant-based burger that satisfies my palate. Unfortunately, many of the most popular plant-based burgers on the market are so filled with ultra-processed ingredients that they don't remotely resemble anything healthy. Since all diet frameworks are invited to the *Eat Smarter* cookout, these real-food plant-based burgers are truly the way to roll.

Combine the broccoli, mushrooms, walnuts, scallions, and cilantro in a food processor. Blend for 1 minute or until the ingredients are all nicely chopped. Add the beans, miso, garlic powder, and cayenne and pulse 10 times for about 3 seconds each time. (You want to break up the beans and mix everything together, but you don't want a completely smooth purée.)

Transfer the mixture to a large bowl and stir in the quinoa flakes. Taste for seasoning and adjust with salt and/or pepper. Form the mixture into eight equal patties.

Heat a large sauté pan over medium-low heat. Add about 1 tablespoon avocado oil and as many burgers as will fit in the pan. (You may need to do this in batches depending on the size of your pan.) Cook for about 5 minutes per side, until the burgers are nicely browned.

Serve in lettuce wraps with avocado and miso mayo.

Serves 4

1 cup broccoli florets (1-inch pieces)

½ pound shiitake mushrooms, stems removed, roughly chopped

½ cup walnut halves and pieces

3 scallions, sliced

⅓ cup chopped fresh cilantro (leaves and stems)

1 (15-ounce) can black beans, rinsed and drained

3 tablespoons white miso

1 teaspoon garlic powder

Pinch of cayenne pepper

1 cup quinoa flakes

Sea salt and black pepper

Avocado oil

8 butter lettuce cups

1 ripe large avocado, pitted, peeled, and sliced

Miso Mayo (page 281)

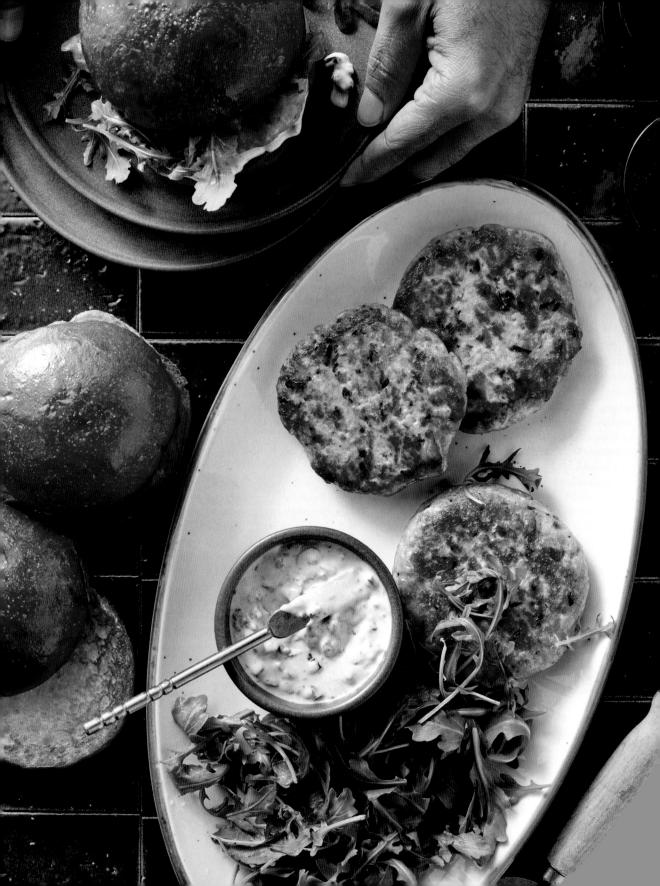

Supreme Salmon Burgers

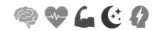

These salmon burgers bring two of the world's favorite foods (salmon and burgers) together in a way that tantalizes your taste buds and fuels your metabolic fire. Serve on buns of your choice, whether it's a gluten-free bun or brioche bun, or it's even delicious in a lettuce wrap. The olive mayo puts this burger into the stratosphere. Make sure your socks are fully secured so that they don't get blown off!

Cut the salmon into 1- to 2-inch chunks and place in the freezer for 15 minutes to firm up.

Meanwhile, make the olive mayo: In a medium bowl, combine the mayo, olives, and lemon juice. Season to taste with sea salt and pepper. Set aside.

When the 15 minutes are up, transfer the salmon to a food processor along with the scallions, lemon, juice, kosher salt, pepper, and mayo. Pulse 3 or 4 times for a couple of seconds each time, until blended but still a bit chunky. Add the breadcrumbs and pulse 1 or 2 more times just to combine everything. Form the mixture into four burgers; if the mixture feels too wet or difficult to work with, add some more breadcrumbs.

Heat a sauté pan over medium heat or heat the grill to medium. Add the burgers and cook for about 5 minutes per side, until nicely browned and cooked through.

Serve the burgers on buns with the olive mayo and arugula.

Serves 4

BURGERS

1½ pounds salmon fillet, skin removed, cut into large chunks

3 scallions (white and light green parts), sliced

Juice of 1 small lemon

1½ teaspoons kosher salt

½ teaspoon black pepper

2 tablespoons of your favorite mayo

¼ cup panko or gluten-free breadcrumbs

OLIVE MAYO

½ cup of your favorite mayo

¼ cup pitted kalamata olives, chopped

Juice of ½ small lemon

Sea salt and black pepper

TO SERVE

4 buns of your choice

2 cups baby arugula

Boss Burgers

When you bite into a great burger, it's like a meditation. It instantly brings you into the present moment, the world slows down around you, and you're transported straight to a blissful inner journey. For this burger patty, itself, it's all about quality ingredients. And from there you get to be the boss on what toppings you choose.

Combine the ground beef, salt, pepper, paprika, garlic powder, onion powder, mustard powder, turmeric, and barbecue sauce in a large bowl. Use your hands to mix gently but thoroughly. Form into four roughly ½-inch-thick burger patties.

Heat a large sauté pan over medium heat or heat the grill to medium. Cook the burgers for 2 to 3 minutes per side for medium rare. Add the cheese slices, turn off the heat and cover with a lid or close the grill for about 30 seconds to quickly melt the cheese.

Transfer the burgers to buns or lettuce leaves, or directly onto a plate. Add toppings of choice. The classic mustard, ketchup, and pickles are fantastic. But lettuce, tomato, onion, avocado slices, and/or spicy mayo are some awesome additions, too!

Serves 4

1 pound $^{80}/_{20}$ ground grass-fed beef

1 teaspoon kosher salt

¼ teaspoon black pepper

½ teaspoon paprika

½ teaspoon garlic powder

½ teaspoon onion powder

½ teaspoon mustard powder

¼ teaspoon ground turmeric

2 tablespoons barbecue sauce

4 slices cheddar cheese

4 buns of your choice, or go animal style and use lettuce leaves (optional)

SUGGESTED TOPPINGS

Mustard

Ketchup

Sliced pickles

Lettuce

Sliced tomato

Sliced ripe avocado

Spicy mayo

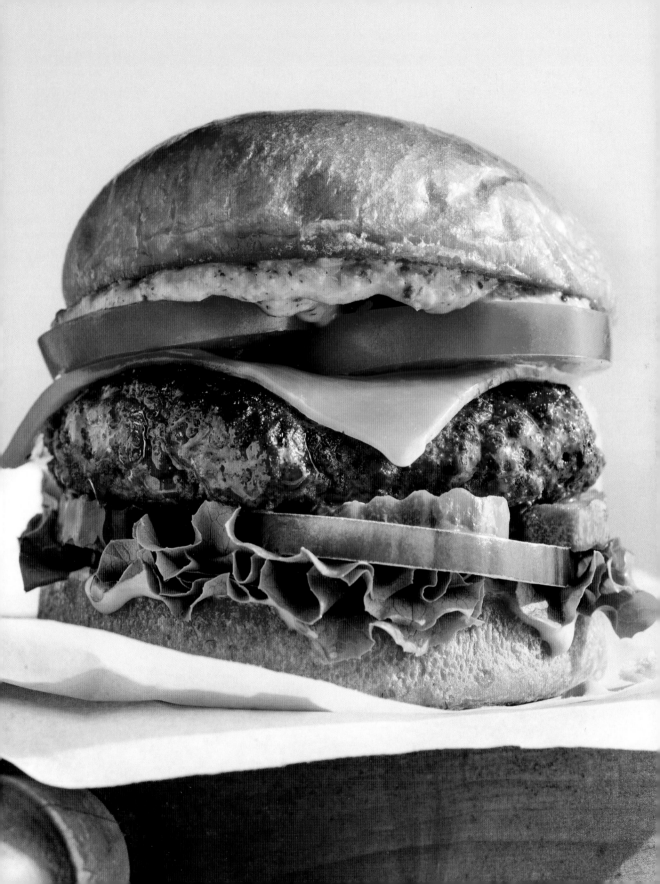

Dinners

CHAPTER EIGHT We dove into all of the remarkable benefits of eating together with family and friends in Chapter One. By scheduling a few family dinners each week, along with delicious recipes like these, you're adding a powerful layer of health and wellness insurance to the people you love. The mission is to take family meals *off* of the endangered list. And the power is in our hands to do it... one meal at a time.

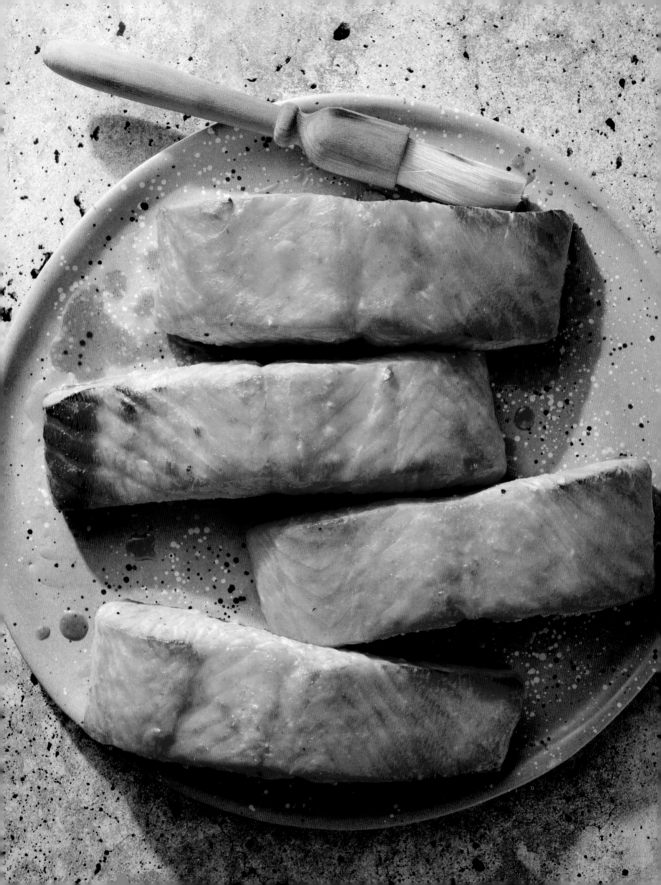

Honey Sriracha Salmon

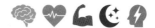

Salmon is the bona fide king of omega-3–rich fatty fish. And the great thing is, you don't have to swim upstream to find mouthwatering recipes to enjoy it. This spicy salmon recipe is one of our family favorites. Keep in mind, cooking time will always depend on the thickness of your fillets. The timing here is based on roughly 1-inch-thick pieces. Serve this with your favorite veggies, such as the ones starting on page 222.

Combine 1 tablespoon of the avocado oil, the sriracha, honey, and salt in a small bowl.

Place the salmon in a shallow bowl, add the hot sauce mixture, and turn to coat the fish. Cover and let marinate for 15 to 20 minutes at room temperature.

Meanwhile, preheat the oven to 425°F. Line a baking sheet with parchment paper.

Transfer the salmon to the baking sheet and roast in the oven for about 12 minutes for medium. If you want a little more color on top, broil for 1 to 2 minutes before removing from the oven.

Plate the salmon and top each fillet with a good squeeze of lemon juice, and an extra dot of sriracha, if you like. Serve and enjoy.

Serves 4

- **2 tablespoons avocado oil**
- **2 tablespoons sriracha hot sauce, plus extra for serving (optional)**
- **2 tablespoons raw honey**
- **½ teaspoon fine sea salt**
- **4 (6- to 8-ounce) skin-on salmon fillets**
- **1 small lemon**

Slow Cooker Chicken Curry

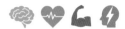

One of my biggest food crushes would have to be curries. I love the spice combinations, nutrient-dense ingredients, and saucy finished products. This chicken curry is a staple at our house. As a little nutrition and flavor bonus, I like to add some kalamata olives on top after it's plated. They actually pair *amazingly* with this dish! Serve with rice or quinoa and a vegetable side of your choice.

Combine the coconut milk, tomato paste, garlic, curry powder, salt, and pepper, in a slow cooker and whisk together. Add the bell peppers and onion, then the chicken. Pour the broth over chicken and mix everything together to completely cover the chicken in the curry mixture.

Cover and cook at low for 6 to 8 hours or high for 4 to 5 hours.

Serves 6

¾ cup unsweetened coconut milk

1 (6-ounce) can tomato paste

3 garlic cloves, minced

4 to 6 tablespoons curry powder (I like lots and use way more than this, but this is a good place to start if you're new to curry)

1½ teaspoons fine sea salt

½ teaspoon black pepper

3 bell peppers (I use yellow and red), cored, seeded, and cut into 1-inch squares

1 yellow onion, thinly sliced

2 pounds boneless skinless chicken, cut into 1- to 2-inch pieces (I use a mix of breasts and thighs)

½ cup chicken broth

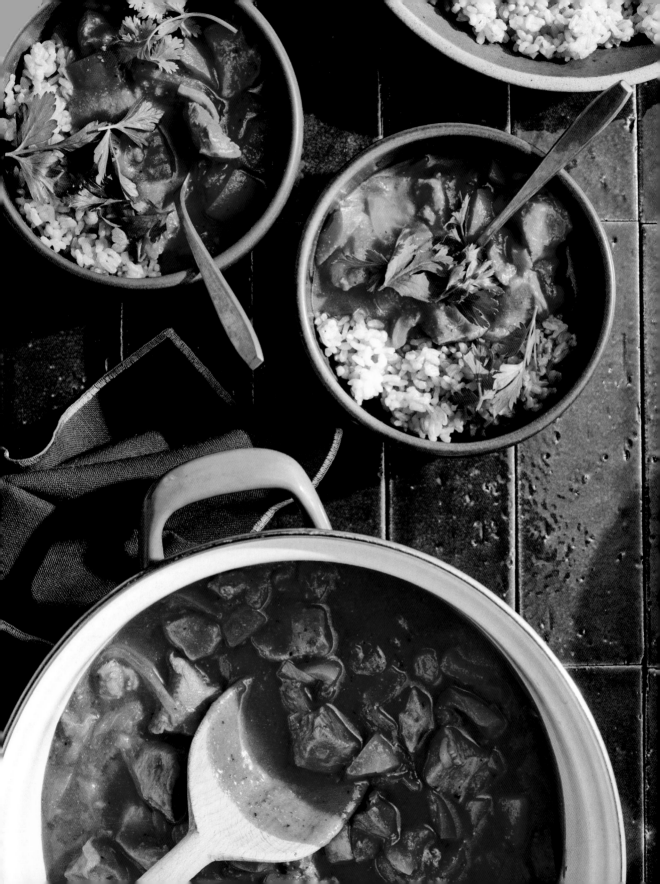

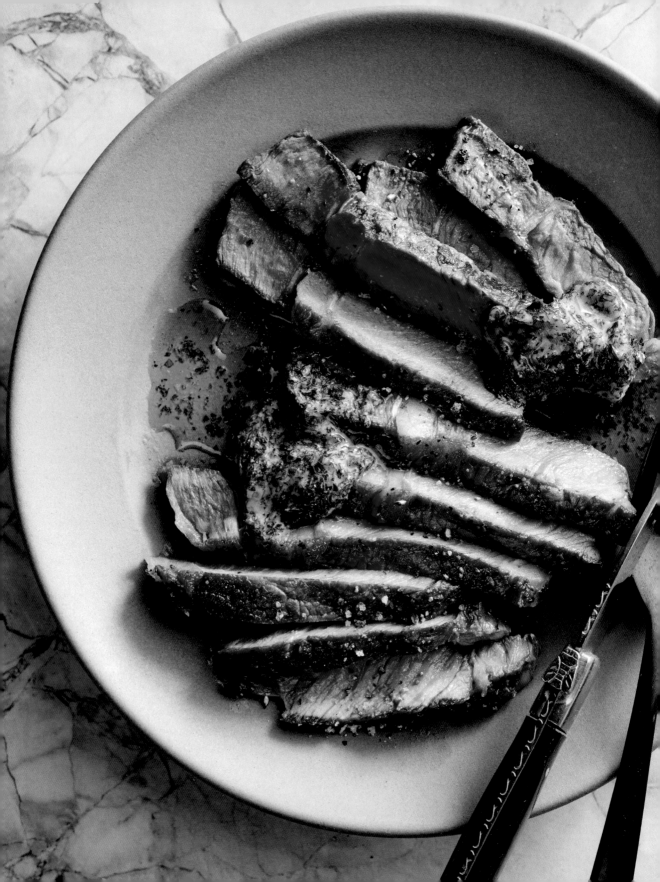

Grilled Steak with Garlic Butter

I highly encourage you to check out the nutritional food facts on grass-fed beef in Chapter Three if you haven't done so already. It's pretty incredible. That said, a lot of people are intimidated about cooking a steak—no one wants to ruin a beautiful piece of meat, especially if it's expensive! But there are a few fundamental tips I've picked up that can make anyone feel like a pro:

Room temp: Take the steak out of the fridge an hour before mealtime so you're not cooking cold meat.

Season ahead: Seasoning steak an hour before you cook it lets the salt permeate the meat to give it lots of flavor.

High heat: Cooking the steak over high heat—whether that's a grill or a cast-iron grill pan—will help amplify the flavor and add a nice crust and grill marks.

Let it rest: Be sure to let the meat rest for at least 5 minutes after pulling it off the heat.

This steak is served with a homemade garlic butter, but you could make it with any sauce, rub, or marinade you like. Serve with your favorite veggies on the side.

To make the garlic butter, mix the butter, ¼ teaspoon of the kosher salt, the minced garlic, garlic powder, and parsley in a small bowl. Transfer to a small piece of plastic wrap, roll into a log, and refrigerate.

Take the steaks out of the fridge 1 hour before you want to cook them. Season evenly with the remaining 2 teaspoons kosher salt, cover, and let sit at room temperature for 1 hour.

Heat the grill or a grill pan to high or medium-high heat. Brush the steaks all over with the avocado oil. Cook, not moving except to flip them once, for about 4 minutes per side for medium-rare. (If you have a meat thermometer, you're looking for an internal temperature of 130°F.) Cook for closer to 3 minutes per side for rare and 5 to 7 minutes for medium to medium-well. Remove the steaks to a large cutting board and let them rest for at least 5 minutes.

Take the garlic butter out of the refrigerator and cut it into 4 slices. Slice the steaks, season with flaky salt, and top with garlic butter.

Serves 4

4 tablespoons unsalted grass-fed butter, softened

2¼ teaspoons kosher salt

1 small garlic clove, minced

¼ teaspoon garlic powder

2 tablespoons finely chopped fresh parsley

2 (1-pound) grass-fed ribeye or NY strip steaks

1 tablespoon avocado oil

Flaky sea salt

Sheet Pan Turmeric Chicken with Sweet Potato and Chickpeas

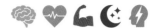

Not only is this recipe jam-packed with ingredients that support metabolic health, this combination was specifically chosen because it's rich in sleep-supporting nutrients as well.

Preheat the oven to 425°F. Line a large baking sheet with parchment paper.

In a large bowl, whisk together the yogurt, 1 teaspoon salt, ½ teaspoon pepper, half of the lemon juice, the turmeric, cumin, paprika, and garlic powder. Toss with the chicken thighs, cover, and let marinate at room temp for at least 10 minutes.

Toss the sweet potato and chickpeas with the olive oil and season with salt and pepper. Arrange them on the baking sheet and add the marinated chicken on top. Roast in the oven for 35 to 40 minutes, until the chicken is cooked through and starting to brown.

Toss the onion with the remaining lemon juice and season with salt and pepper. Garnish the chicken with the onion salad and cilantro leaves before serving.

Note: If you can, go for chicken thighs that are on the smaller side to make sure the sheet pan doesn't get too crowded.

Serves 4 to 6

½ cup grass-fed whole milk Greek yogurt

Kosher salt and black pepper

Juice of 1 lemon

½ teaspoon ground turmeric

½ teaspoon ground cumin

½ teaspoon paprika

½ teaspoon garlic powder

6 boneless skinless chicken thighs (about 1¼ pounds total; see Note)

1 medium sweet potato, scrubbed and cut into roughly ½-inch chunks

1 (15-ounce) can chickpeas, rinsed and drained

2 tablespoons olive oil

¼ red onion, thinly sliced

¼ cup roughly chopped fresh cilantro leaves

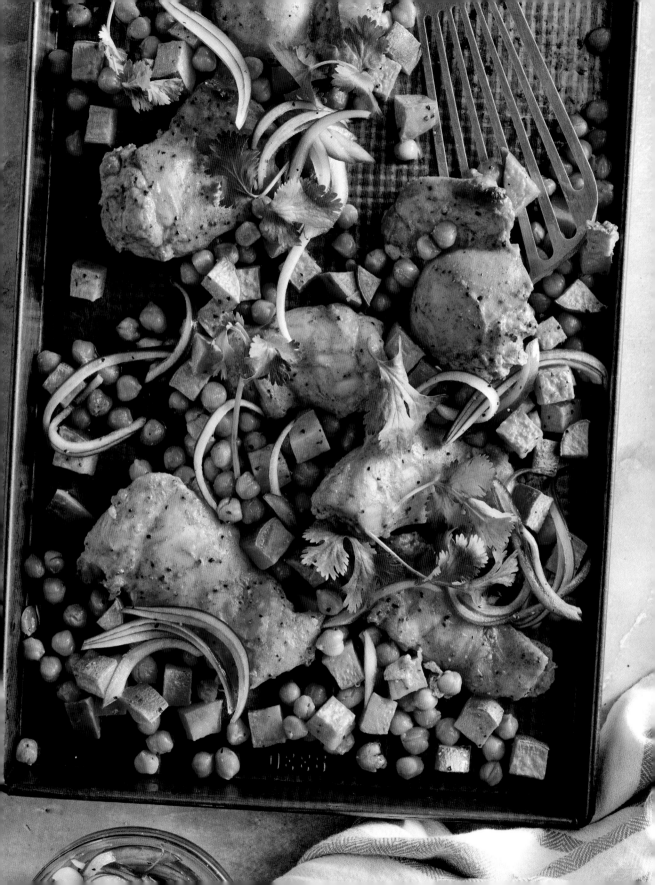

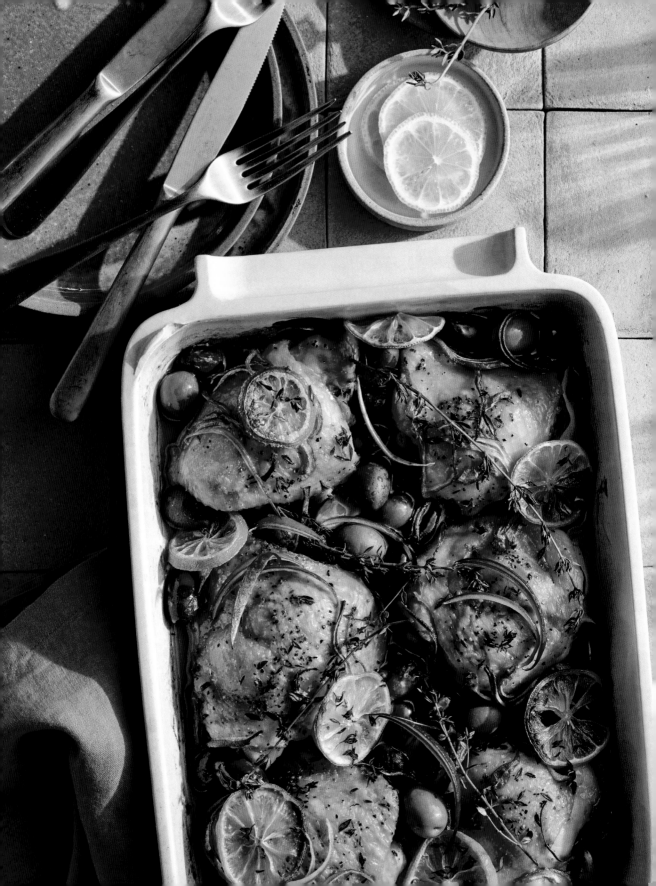

Oven-Roasted Chicken Thighs with Olives

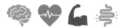

It's not a coincidence that olives are highlighted in so many ancient texts and even carved into the pyramids of pharaohs. There's something truly special about this food that, today, modern science is beginning to uncover. Olives are rich in vital fats and provide a wealth of prebiotic benefits. Plus, they're an absolute treasure trove of antioxidants. You can use whatever mix of olives you like for this bountiful dish—we often use a mix of kalamata and Castelvetrano. Be sure to serve this with rice, cauliflower rice, or some other grain or pasta to soak up all of the delicious sauce in the baking dish!

Preheat oven to 375°F

Put the chicken thighs in a large (9 by 13-inch or similar) baking dish. (You want them to be relatively snug but not overlapping at all.) Season generously with salt and pepper, then toss with the onion, lemon, olives, garlic, thyme, and olive oil. Cover and let marinate at room temp for 30 minutes.

Uncover, add the water, and cook in the oven for 1 hour to 1 hour 15 minutes, until the skin is nicely browned.

Serves 4 to 6

6 bone-in skinless chicken thighs (about 2 pounds total)

Sea salt and black pepper

½ red onion, thinly sliced

1 lemon, sliced

¾ cup mixed pitted olives

4 large garlic cloves, smashed and peeled

1 tablespoon fresh thyme leaves

3 tablespoons olive oil

½ cup water

Blackened Shrimp Kebabs

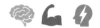

These simple kebabs pack a nutritional punch and are so full of flavor! Serve these as an appetizer, on a grain bowl, or as part of a mixed grill dinner with Grilled Zucchini and Peppers (page 197) and Easy Quinoa and Cauliflower "Pilaf" (page 234). You can whip these kebabs up on the grill, but they're also great seared in a hot cast-iron pan. Time-saving tip: Double or triple this spice blend and keep it on hand to use on chicken, steak, or veggies!

If you're using wooden skewers, soak them in water for at least 20 minutes.

Combine the garlic powder, onion powder, thyme, paprika, cayenne, sugar, black pepper, and salt in a large bowl. Add the olive oil and shrimp, mix well, and marinate for at least 10 minutes at room temp. Or cover and marinate up to overnight in the fridge.

Heat the grill to medium-high and divide the shrimp between the skewers. Grill for 2 to 3 minutes per side, until the shrimp have nice grill marks and are pink all the way through.

Serves 4

8 wooden or metal skewers

½ teaspoon garlic powder

½ teaspoon onion powder

½ teaspoon dried thyme

½ teaspoon paprika

¼ teaspoon cayenne pepper

½ teaspoon coconut sugar

¼ teaspoon black pepper

¾ teaspoon fine sea salt

2 tablespoons olive oil

1 pound peeled large shrimp

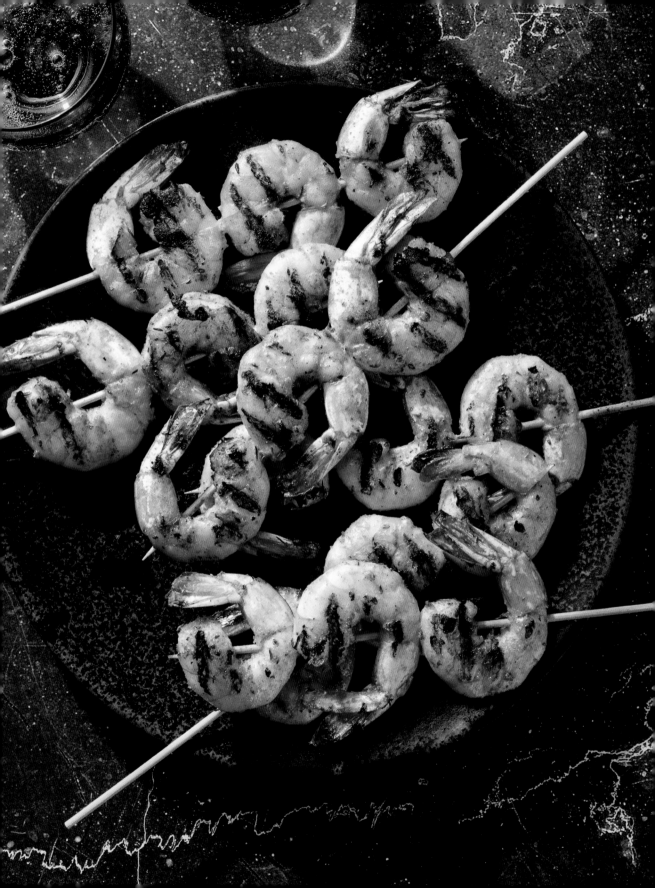

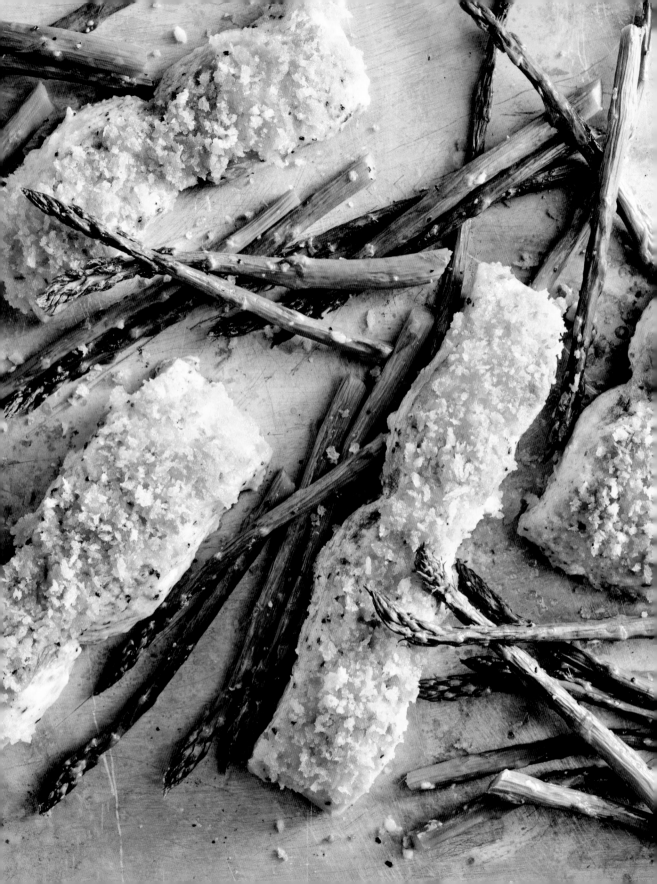

Sheet Pan Fish with Mayo-Lemon Sauce and Asparagus

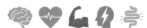

The first time I had mahi mahi was one of the greatest moments of my life. My wife (then girlfriend) took me—at the age of 25— on my very first flight, to Miami, Florida. I'd never seen the ocean before, let alone experienced a meal by the beach. It was an absolute feast for my senses. The savory, creamy fish, the boundless ocean reaching out past the horizon, and my best friend there with me to experience it all. I wanted to create a dish reminiscent of that moment, and I think you're going to love it.

Preheat the oven to 425°F. Line a large baking sheet with parchment paper.

Arrange the asparagus on one side of the baking sheet and the fish fillets on the other.

Season the fish generously with salt and pepper and squeeze over the juice from half of the lemon. Season the asparagus with salt and pepper and toss with 1 tablespoon of the olive oil.

In a small bowl, mix the mayo, onion powder, garlic powder, and cayenne. In another small bowl, mix the breadcrumbs and the remaining olive oil and season with a pinch of salt. Top each fillet with about 1 tablespoon of the mayo mixture, then sprinkle over the breadcrumbs.

Transfer to the oven and cook for about 12 minutes, until the fish is cooked through and the breadcrumbs are just starting to brown.

Squeeze over the remaining lemon juice and serve immediately.

Note: This recipe includes panko breadcrumbs. If you're avoiding gluten, simply swap in gluten-free breadcrumbs instead. We like Ian's.

Serves 4

- **1 bunch asparagus, woody ends removed**
- **4 (6-ounce) mahi mahi or any white fish fillets**
- **Sea salt and black pepper**
- **1 lemon, cut in half**
- **2 tablespoons olive oil**
- **¼ cup of your favorite mayo**
- **½ teaspoon onion powder**
- **½ teaspoon garlic powder**
- **Pinch of cayenne pepper**
- **¼ cup panko or gluten-free breadcrumbs (see Note)**

White Fish with Kelp Butter

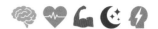

This delightful combination of white fish and the nutrient-rich sea veggie kelp is reminiscent of a dish you'd enjoy at an expensive French restaurant. Yet it's quick to throw together and actually very budget-friendly. I'd recommend serving this with a side salad and an approved, smarter grain of choice to bring everything together.

To make the kelp butter, combine the softened butter and kelp flakes in a small bowl. Use a fork to mix and set aside.

Season the fish with salt and pepper on both sides. Heat a large sauté pan over medium heat. While the pan heats up, place the flour in a shallow bowl and lightly dredge the fish pieces all over.

Add the avocado oil to the pan. Shake the fish to get rid of any extra flour and cook for about 2 minutes per side, until just firm to the touch.

Add the kelp butter and let it bubble and foam for a few seconds while swirling the pan. When it is just starting to brown, add the lemon juice and turn off the heat.

Transfer the fish to plates, pour over the kelp butter sauce, and serve with lemon wedges on the side.

Serves 4

4 tablespoons unsalted grass-fed butter, slightly softened

1 teaspoon kelp flakes

4 (6-ounce) mild white fish fillets (such as cod or halibut, about ¾-inch thick), skin removed

Sea salt and black pepper

¼ cup all-purpose or gluten-free flour

1 to 2 tablespoons avocado oil

Juice of 1 small lemon

Lemon wedges

Bacon-Wrapped Chicken Tenders

Rather than a run-of-the-mill cold cuts sandwich, we often make these tasty tenders for my youngest son to take for school lunches. Along with a dipping sauce, some fresh fruit, and another little treat, it's a protein-powered real-food lunch that kids enjoy. These also work as great appetizers when you have company over for game night or a sporting event.

Preheat the oven to 400°F. Line a baking sheet with foil and place a wire rack on top of it.

Mix the onion powder, garlic powder, paprika, chili powder, salt, and pepper in a small bowl.

Working in batches, lay out the bacon on a cutting board between two pieces of parchment paper and use a heavy pan to pound it into thinner strips. (This will help them wrap all the way around the tenders and crisp up in the oven.)

Season the chicken tenders with half of the spice mix, then wrap each one with a piece of bacon. Place on the wire rack and season with the remaining spice mix.

Transfer to the oven and cook for 15 minutes. Turn the heat up to 450°F and cook for another 10 to 15 minutes, until the bacon is starting to crisp up. Remove from the oven and allow them to cool. Serve or pack away in a safe travel container for school lunch.

Serves 4 to 6

1 teaspoon onion powder

1 teaspoon garlic powder

1 teaspoon paprika

1 teaspoon chili powder

½ teaspoon kosher salt

½ teaspoon black pepper

6 slices bacon, cut in half crosswise

12 chicken tenders, or 2 large boneless skinless chicken breasts, cut into 6 strips each

Chicken Crust Pizza Two Ways

When I was a kid, having the chance to order a pizza was cause for celebration. Over the years, I've tried to find creative ways to upgrade one of my favorite family food experiences, and this recipe is the result. Not only is this pizza a protein powerhouse, it's gluten-free, keto-friendly, and checks a lot of extra boxes for health-minded shoppers today. This recipe makes two thin crusts. Keep in mind, it's not as firm as a typical thin crust pizza, but it gets the job done in a delicious and nutritious way. If you aren't making two pizzas, simply freeze the second raw crust or bake it off and freeze the cooked base so it's ready to be topped and quickly baked in the oven whenever you're craving it.

CHICKEN PIZZA CRUST

Preheat the oven to 400°F.

Mix the chicken, salt, onion powder, garlic powder, parmesan, and egg together in a large bowl.

Divide into two equal portions. Place one on a large sheet of parchment paper. Top with another large sheet of parchment and use a rolling pin to carefully roll the base into a very thin (about ⅛-inch), slightly oblong shape. (It doesn't have to be perfect but does need to fit on your baking sheet!) Slide the crust, still between the parchment sheets, onto a large baking sheet, then carefully peel off the top layer of parchment.

Transfer to the oven and cook for 20 to 25 minutes, until the crust is cooked through and starting to brown in places.

Your chicken pizza is now ready to be topped and cooked. Use immediately or cool and store in the fridge for up to 2 days or tightly wrapped in the freezer for up to 3 months.

Makes 2 crusts

- **1 pound ground chicken (preferably dark meat)**
- **1 teaspoon kosher salt**
- **½ teaspoon onion powder**
- **½ teaspoon garlic powder**
- **⅔ cup lightly packed finely grated parmesan cheese**
- **1 large organic egg**

No. 1
Chicken Parm Pizza

This version gives me the vibes of the classic pizza I love!

Serves 2 to 4

½ recipe Chicken Pizza Crust, rolled out and baked

3 tablespoons marinara sauce or crushed jarred tomatoes

2 ounces fresh mozzarella cheese, sliced or torn into large pieces

¼ cup grated parmesan cheese

Fresh basil leaves, torn

Heat the broiler.

Carefully slide the pizza crust off of the parchment paper directly onto the baking sheet. (This is to keep from burning the parchment under the broiler.) Top the crust evenly with the marinara sauce, mozzarella, and parm. Broil for about 5 minutes, until the cheese are bubbling and starting to brown. Garnish with basil and enjoy!

No. 2
Cauliflower Buffalo Pizza

Just one bite of this pizza, and it will very likely become a staple for game days and Super Bowl parties for years to come!

Serves 2 to 4

½ recipe Chicken Pizza Crust

3 slices bacon, diced

1 tablespoon olive oil

½ medium head cauliflower, broken into small florets and roughly chopped

Sea salt and black pepper

2 tablespoons Smarter Ranch Dressing (page 286) or your favorite store-bought ranch dressing

2 tablespoons Frank's RedHot sauce

1 scallion, thinly sliced

Roll out and cook the pizza crust according to the main recipe. While the crust bakes, heat a medium sauté pan over medium heat. Add the bacon and cook for about 2 minutes, until it's starting to crisp up.

Add the olive oil and cauliflower, season with a little salt and pepper, and cook for another 5 minutes, until the cauliflower is tender and starting to brown.

Mix the ranch dressing and hot sauce in a small bowl.

When the crust is done, take it out of the oven but leave the oven on. Spread on half of the ranch dressing mixture, top with the bacon and cauliflower, then drizzle over the remaining dressing. Pop the pizza back in the oven for 5 minutes until the toppings are hot. Garnish with the scallion and serve.

Bangers and Mash with Sauerkraut

I feel a huge connection to the incredible listeners of my show who are based in the U.K. We obviously share some cultural similarities, both being western nations, but there are a wide variety of differences to appreciate as well—in particular when it comes to traditional food items. When I first heard the name "bangers and mash", I knew that I had to try it! It's become one of my favorite dishes, and with this healthier spin to the classic British pub dish, it'll likely become one of your favorites as well.

Preheat the oven to 375°F.

Heat a 10-inch ovenproof skillet over medium-high heat. Add 1 tablespoon of the avocado oil and sear the sausages for about 2 minutes per side, until nicely browned. Remove to a plate.

Add the remaining tablespoon avocado oil, the onion, garlic, thyme, and a generous pinch each of salt and black pepper. Turn the heat down to medium and cook, stirring every so often, for about 5 minutes, until the onion is softened.

Add ¼ cup of the water to the pan and use a wooden spoon to scrape up any browned bits on the bottom of the pan. Cook off the liquid, then nestle in the sausages, making sure to move the onions around so the sausages are touching the pan. (This will help them brown more as they cook.)

Transfer the pan to the oven and roast for 20 minutes or until the sausages are fully cooked.

continues

Serves 4

- 2 tablespoons avocado oil
- 4 pork, turkey, or chicken bratwurst sausages (about 1½ pounds total)
- 1 medium yellow onion, thinly sliced
- 2 garlic cloves, thinly sliced
- ½ teaspoon dried thyme
- Sea salt and black pepper
- 1 cup water or chicken broth
- 1 pound potatoes (I use a mix of russet and Yukon gold), peeled and cut into 1-inch dice
- ½ medium head cauliflower, cut into 2-inch pieces
- 4 tablespoons unsalted grass-fed butter
- 1 tablespoon all-purpose or gluten-free flour
- 1 to 2 cups sauerkraut

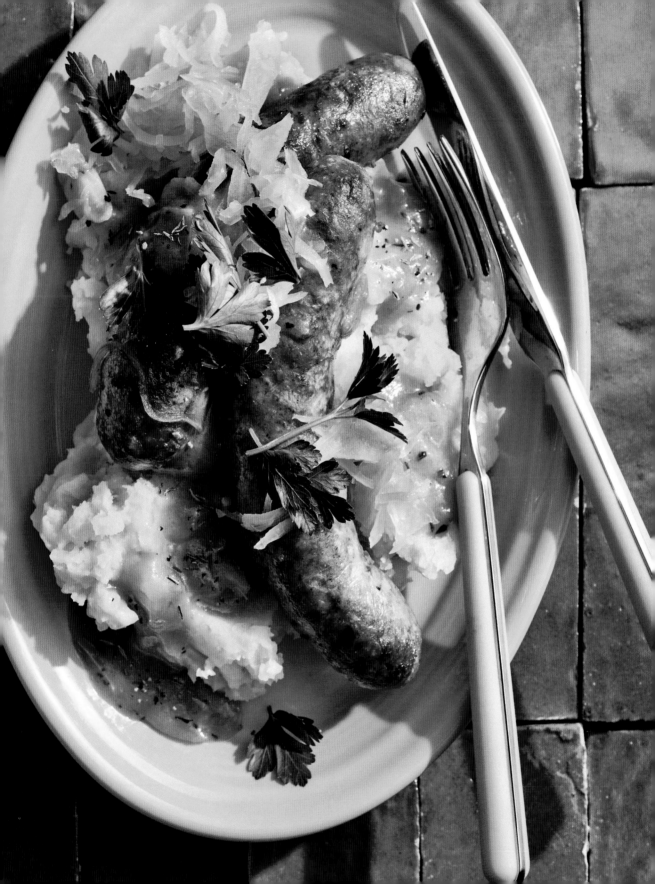

Meanwhile, place the potatoes in a medium pot with lots of salted water and bring up to a boil. Add the cauliflower, reduce to a simmer, and cook for about 10 minutes, until the potatoes can be easily pierced with a fork or knife. Drain, then return to the pot. Mash with a potato masher. Stir in 3 tablespoons of the butter and season to taste with salt and pepper. Cover to keep warm.

Carefully remove the pan from the oven and transfer the sausages to a plate. Put the pan over medium heat and add the remaining tablespoon butter. When the butter has melted, add the flour and cook for 1 minute, stirring constantly with a wooden spoon. Pour in the remaining ¾ cup water and cook, stirring, for 2 to 3 minutes, until the sauce has thickened into a nice gravy. Season to taste with salt and pepper.

Divide the potato-cauliflower mash between four plates, top each with a sausage, and pour over the onion gravy. Serve with lots of sauerkraut on the side.

Stuffed Sweet Potatoes

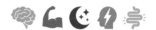

Simple, nutrient-rich, and scrumptious. These stuffed sweet potatoes are the base model for a limitless variety of additional toppings you can feel free to add. Olives, avocado, hemp seeds—the list goes on and on. I recommend serving with a healthy portion of your favorite veggies as well. We love steamed broccoli or roasted Brussels sprouts as a healthy pairing with this dish.

Preheat the oven to 400°F. Line a baking sheet with parchment paper or foil.

Place sweet potatoes on the baking sheet and cook for 1 hour.

When the potatoes have cooked for about 45 minutes, heat a large skillet over medium heat and add the ground beef. Sauté for about 5 minutes, breaking it up with a spatula or wooden spoon, until the meat is starting to brown and is nearly cooked through. Stir in the salt, pepper, paprika, garlic powder, onion powder, mustard, and turmeric. Mix in thoroughly, cover, and let simmer for a few more minutes.

Take the sweet potatoes out of the oven, let them cool for a few minutes, then slice them open lengthwise and slather with 1 tablespoon butter each. Top each sweet potato with the ground beef mixture and additional toppings of your choice.

Serves 4

4 medium sweet potatoes (Japanese, if possible!), scrubbed

1 pound 80/20 ground grass-fed beef

1 teaspoon kosher salt

¼ teaspoon black pepper

½ teaspoon paprika

½ teaspoon garlic powder

½ teaspoon onion powder

½ teaspoon mustard powder

¼ teaspoon ground turmeric

4 tablespoons unsalted grass-fed butter, slightly softened

Additional toppings, such as olives, avocado, or hemp seeds

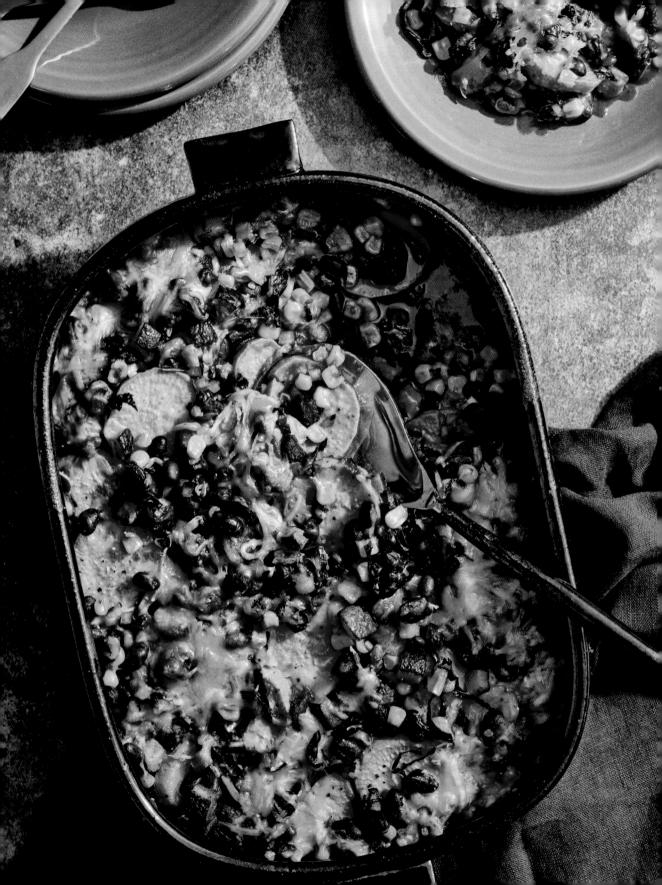

Sweet Potato Enchilada Casserole

Here's a healthier twist on a house favorite. This is a fantastic vegetarian meal, but you could definitely add a layer of shredded rotisserie chicken or sautéed ground beef to up the protein. It's beyond delicious on its own, but my family usually takes it up a notch and serves it with sliced avocado, pickled jalapeños, fresh cilantro, sour cream, sliced olives, and hot sauce on the side. Endless possibilities!

Preheat the oven to 425°F. Line a baking sheet with parchment paper.

Peel and slice the sweet potatoes about ⅓-inch thick. Toss with 1 tablespoon of the olive oil and season with salt and pepper. Arrange the slices on the baking sheet. Roast for 30 minutes or until tender and starting to brown.

Heat a large sauté pan over medium-high heat. Add the remaining 2 tablespoons olive oil, then stir in the zucchini, kale, and corn. Season with salt and pepper and sauté for 3 to 5 minutes, stirring often to make sure nothing is sticking to the pan, until the zucchini is tender and the kale has cooked down. Add the garlic powder, cumin, and ground chipotle and cook for another 1 to 2 minutes.

Transfer the veggies to a large bowl. Stir in the beans and onion. Season to taste with salt and pepper.

Remove the sweet potatoes from the oven and turn the oven down to 400°F. Spoon one-third of the salsa into a 9 by 13-inch (or similar) baking dish. Layer in half of the sweet potatoes, half of the bean and veggie mixture, another third of the salsa, and half of the cheese. Repeat the process, starting with the sweet potatoes and finishing with the remaining cheese.

Bake uncovered for 20 to 25 minutes, until the casserole is bubbling and smells amazing.

Finish under the broiler for 1 to 2 minutes for a crispy cheese topping.

Serves 6

- **2 large or 3 medium sweet potatoes**
- **3 tablespoons olive oil**
- **Sea salt and black pepper**
- **1 medium zucchini, diced (about 1½ cups)**
- **½ bunch lacinato kale (aka dino kale), ribs removed, thinly sliced**
- **1 cup frozen corn kernels**
- **½ teaspoon garlic powder**
- **½ teaspoon ground cumin**
- **¼ teaspoon ground chipotle**
- **1 (15-ounce) can black beans, rinsed and drained**
- **¼ cup finely diced red onion**
- **1 (15-ounce) jar your favorite salsa or enchilada sauce**
- **8 ounces shredded cheddar or Mexican blend cheese (2 cups)**

Stuffed Bell Peppers

My favorite thing about these stuffed peppers is that they come wrapped in a bowl you get to eat! Of course, we've got the metabolism-supportive nutrients of the grass-fed beef. And if you'd like to make it a lower-carb meal, you can opt to use cauliflower rice instead of standard rice here. Just cook your cauliflower rice for 5 minutes before adding to the beef mixture.

Preheat the oven to 350°F.

Cut off the tops of the peppers. Discard seeds and membranes. Chop enough of the tops to make ¼ cup; set aside.

Bring a large pot of water up to a boil, add the cleaned peppers, and cook, uncovered, for about 5 minutes, until the peppers are tender but not soft.

Remove the peppers with tongs or a slotted spoon and invert them onto a plate lined with paper towels or a dish towel to drain well.

Sprinkle the insides of the peppers lightly with salt.

Heat a large skillet over medium-high heat. Add the ground beef, onion, and reserved chopped bell pepper and sauté, stirring often, until the meat is browned and vegetables are tender. Carefully drain off any excess fat.

Add the tomatoes, 1 teaspoon salt, the Worcestershire, paprika, spinach, and ½ teaspoon pepper to the skillet and cook for another minute or two.

Transfer the meat mixture to a large bowl and stir in the rice and almost all of the cheese. (I like to reserve a few tablespoons to sprinkle over the top.) Stuff the peppers with meat mixture and place in a baking dish that will hold them snugly. Cover with foil and bake for 25 minutes, until bubbling.

Remove the foil, sprinkle with the reserved cheese, and bake for 5 more minutes, until the cheese is nicely melted.

Serves 4

4 large red or yellow bell peppers

Kosher salt and black pepper

1 pound 80/20 ground grass-fed beef or other ground meat of your choice

½ cup chopped red or yellow onion

1 (16-ounce) can diced tomatoes, drained

1 teaspoon Worcestershire sauce

1 teaspoon paprika

1 cup baby spinach firmly packed, roughly chopped

1½ cups cooked white or brown rice

½ cup shredded cheddar cheese

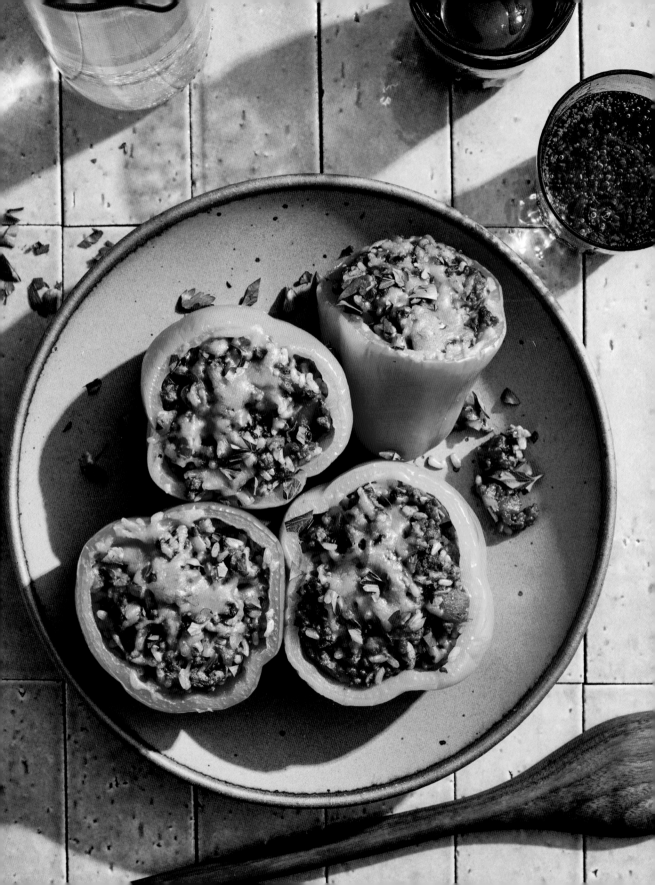

Salisbury Steak Meatballs

When my wife told me she was making Salisbury steak meatballs, my mind transported back to the sad TV dinners my siblings and I had growing up in the '80s and '90s. Suffice it to say, these real-food meatballs have revolutionized my ideas of what Salisbury steak can be. They're so good! And it's one of our go-to foods for food prep to reheat and eat throughout the week. I highly recommend serving with a smarter-approved grain of choice and sauerkraut.

Finely chop 1 ounce of the mushrooms into small pieces and set aside.

Heat a large, safe nonstick sauté pan over medium-high heat. Add 2 tablespoons of the oil and the onions and cook until golden brown, 4 to 5 minutes.

In a large bowl, combine half of the sautéed onions with the ground beef, ground turkey, chopped mushrooms, breadcrumbs, egg, 1 tablespoon of the tomato paste, ¼ cup of the beef broth, 1 teaspoon salt, and 1 teaspoon black pepper.

In a small bowl, whisk together the flour and the rest of the broth. Mix in remaining onions, remaining tomato paste, vinegar, the Worcestershire sauce, and mustard powder and whisk until smooth. Set aside.

Roll the meat mixture into 20 small meatballs. Turn the heat to medium-high, add the remaining 2 tablespoons oil, and brown the meatballs for about 2 minutes per side, until nicely browned and no longer sticking to the pan.

Transfer meatballs to a slow cooker. Stir in the sauce and the remaining sliced mushrooms. Season with a little salt and pepper, cover, and cook on low heat for 6 to 8 hours, until the sauce has thickened slightly and the meatballs are very tender.

Serve with a sprinkling of parsley, if you like.

Serves 4

- **5 ounces sliced cremini mushrooms**
- **4 tablespoons avocado oil**
- **½ yellow onion, minced**
- **½ pound 93% lean ground grass-fed beef**
- **½ pound 93% lean ground turkey**
- **⅓ cup panko or gluten-free breadcrumbs**
- **1 large organic egg, beaten**
- **2 tablespoons tomato paste**
- **1¼ cups reduced-sodium beef broth or Beef Bone Broth (page 173)**
- **Kosher salt and black pepper**
- **1 tablespoon all-purpose or gluten-free flour**
- **1 teaspoon white wine vinegar**
- **2 teaspoons Worcestershire sauce**
- **¼ teaspoon mustard powder**
- **Chopped fresh parsley (optional)**

Beef Stew

This wholesome classic has been upgraded with high-quality ingredients. It makes for a wonderful family dinner, as well as a hearty lunch if you make enough for leftovers. We used a slow cooker here, but we've found great (and speedy) success using an Instant Pot from time to time, too. Serve with white rice and your favorite green veggie on the side—the Brain-Boosting Garlicky Spinach (page 241) or Steamed Broccoli (page 225) are favorites at our house!

Put the beef, flour, and 1½ teaspoons salt in a resealable bag. Seal the bag and shake until the meat is nicely coated.

Heat a large Dutch oven over medium-high heat. Add 2 tablespoons of the avocado oil and let sizzle. Add the coated meat, shaking off any excess flour, and cook until browned on all sides. (You may need to add a little more oil as the meat cooks to keep any flour from burning on the bottom of the pot.) Transfer the meat to the slow cooker.

Add the remaining avocado oil and the onion to the pot and sauté for 3 to 5 minutes, using a wooden spoon to stir and scrape up any brown bits on the bottom of the pot. When the onions are translucent, add the garlic and sauté for 1 more minute.

Add the tomato paste, stir for 1 minute, then pour in the beef broth. Cook for another minute or so, using your wooden spoon to scrape up any brown bits.

Carefully pour the onion mixture into the slow cooker. Add the carrots, potatoes, Worcestershire sauce, Italian seasoning, paprika, ½ teaspoon salt, and ½ teaspoon black pepper. Cover and cook on low for 8 hours.

Season with more salt and pepper to taste before serving.

Serves 4 to 6

- **1½ pounds grass-fed beef chuck or stew meat, cut into 1- to 2-inch dice**
- **¼ cup all-purpose or gluten free flour**
- **Kosher salt and black pepper**
- **4 tablespoons avocado oil**
- **½ yellow onion, chopped**
- **2 garlic cloves, minced**
- **2 tablespoons no-salt-added tomato paste**
- **1½ cups reduced-sodium beef broth or Beef Bone Broth (page 173)**
- **3 carrots, chopped**
- **3 or 4 small organic red potatoes (about ½ pound total), quartered**
- **1 tablespoon Worcestershire sauce.**
- **1 teaspoon Italian seasoning**
- **1 teaspoon paprika**

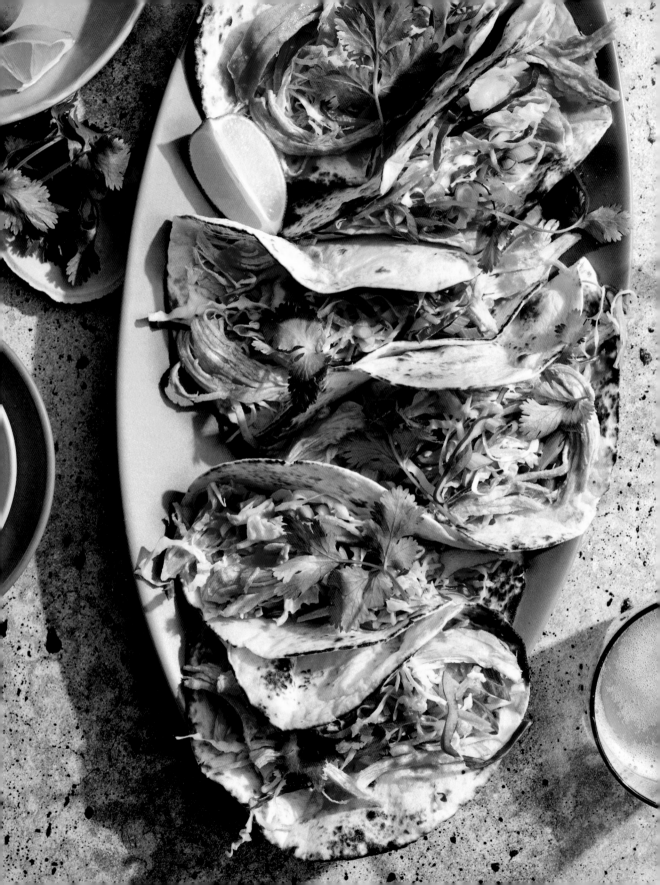

Buffalo Chicken Tacos

At our house, we're often doing Taco Tuesdays or Fiesta Fridays with traditional tacos, burrito bowls, or this spicy spin that delivers serious enjoyment. This is one you have to taste to believe. I guarantee you'll be blown away!

Combine the butter, hot sauce, garlic powder, and onion powder in a bowl and mix well. (Works great with just butter and hot sauce as well.)

Line the bottom of the slow cooker with the chicken breasts. Season with salt and pepper.

Pour the hot sauce mixture over chicken and turn the breasts to coat evenly. Place the lid on the slow cooker, set on high, and cook for 4 hours.

Once cooked, shred the chicken in the slow cooker using two forks.

Whisk together the honey and vinegar in a small bowl. Add the mayo, whisk to combine, then slowly whisk in the olive oil. Season to taste with salt and pepper and set aside. Put the coleslaw mix in a serving bowl and add the scallions and cilantro. Toss with the dressing and season to taste with more salt and pepper, if desired.

To serve, fill the tortillas with the chicken. (*Important*: Use tongs or a slotted spoon to let some of the liquid drain off.) Top with coleslaw and enjoy!

Serves 4

- ½ cup or 8 tablespoons (1 stick) unsalted grass-fed butter, melted
- ½ cup Frank's RedHot sauce or another comparable brand
- 2 teaspoons garlic powder
- 1 teaspoon onion powder
- 4 boneless skinless chicken breasts (about 2 pounds total)
- Sea salt and black pepper
- ½ teaspoon raw honey
- 1 tablespoon apple cider vinegar
- 1 tablespoon of your favorite mayo
- 3 tablespoons olive oil
- 1 (12-ounce) bag organic coleslaw mix
- 2 scallions, thinly sliced
- ¼ cup chopped fresh cilantro
- 8 medium flour tortillas or your favorite gluten-free tortillas

Veggies
& Sides

CHAPTER NINE   Many of the greatest superheroes have talented companions at their side. These nourishing dishes provide a perfect sidekick to the powerhouse main courses in the *Eat Smarter Family Cookbook*.

Sautéed Curry Cabbage

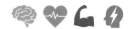

Have you ever thought about how a head of cabbage can look similar to what's hiding away in our own heads? In a randomized controlled trial, published in the *Journal of Nutrition*, this reminiscently dual-hemisphered vegetable was found to reduce biomarkers of inflammation that protect our brains and cardiovascular system. Combined with the power of turmeric, you've got a truly special brain-boosting tandem.[11]

Heat the coconut oil in a large skillet over medium heat. Add the onion and cook until it begins to soften. Add the cabbage and cook for a few minutes, tossing occasionally to be sure all sides are lightly cooked. Add the curry powder, mustard (if using), and salt, mix thoroughly, then mix in the water.

Cover and reduce the heat to medium-low. Simmer, stirring occasionally, for 10 to 15 minutes, until soft but not mushy!

Sprinkle the kelp on top just before serving, if using.

Serves 2

1 tablespoon coconut oil

⅓ cup chopped white onion

½ medium head green cabbage, shredded

1 tablespoon curry powder

1 teaspoon mustard powder (optional, but good!)

2 pinches of fine sea salt

¼ cup water

1 teaspoon kelp granules (optional)

Steamed Broccoli with Grass-Fed Butter

When I think of fresh steamed broccoli, I think of the home-cooked meals my grandmother would make for me. One of my proudest moments was when she made the fish my grandfather and I had just caught, potatoes, and some buttery steamed broccoli. Today, it's a staple in our house. It's simple, fresh, and pairs well with a variety of meals.

Cut any large florets in half so all of the pieces of broccoli are roughly the same size.

Put the butter and garlic powder in a small bowl or ramekin and use a fork to mix.

Combine the garlic butter, broccoli, water, salt, and pepper in a Dutch oven or similar pan wide enough to fit all of the broccoli in one layer. Turn on the heat to medium-high. When the water is just beginning to steam and the butter is starting to sizzle, cover the pot, turn the heat down to low or medium-low (you want to maintain a steady simmer), and cook for 8 to 10 minutes, until tender.

Transfer to a serving dish and enjoy!

Serves 4

1 large head broccoli, cut into florets (about 6 cups)

2 tablespoons unsalted grass-fed butter, slightly softened

1 teaspoon garlic powder

¼ cup water

½ teaspoon kosher salt

¼ teaspoon black pepper

Roasted Artichoke Hearts with Garlic and Parmesan

Artichokes provide some of the most notable prebiotic benefits ever discovered. For instance, a double-blind placebo-controlled study cited in the *British Journal of Nutrition* revealed that compounds contained in artichokes have a "pronounced prebiotic effect" and help improve the ratios of friendly flora in our microbiome. Artichokes are awesome, but they can be intimidating and time-consuming to work with when they're fresh. Instead, using frozen artichokes (which are preserved at the peak of freshness) makes them an easy, affordable, good-for-you side dish you can enjoy year-round. Of course, you can have this dish as a side along with dinner, but they also make a great appetizer with our Smarter Ranch Dressing (page 286) for dipping![12]

Preheat the oven to 425°F. Line a large baking sheet with parchment paper.

Drain the artichoke hearts in a colander, gently pressing to release any liquid without breaking them up. Transfer to a dish towel or paper towels and press gently with another cloth or more paper towels on top to dry out even more.

Put the artichokes in a large bowl and toss with the olive oil, garlic, onion powder, and season generously with salt and pepper.

Transfer to the baking sheet and spread out in a single layer. Roast for 25 minutes or until golden and crispy.

Pull the baking sheet out, top the artichokes with the parm, and return them to the oven for 3 to 5 minutes, until the artichokes are crispy and the cheese is starting to brown.

Serve hot with lemon wedges on the side.

Serves 4

- **2 (12-ounce) bags frozen quartered artichoke hearts, thawed overnight in the fridge**
- **2 tablespoons olive oil**
- **2 large garlic cloves, minced**
- **1 teaspoon onion powder**
- **Sea salt and black pepper**
- **¼ cup finely grated parmesan cheese**
- **Lemon wedges**

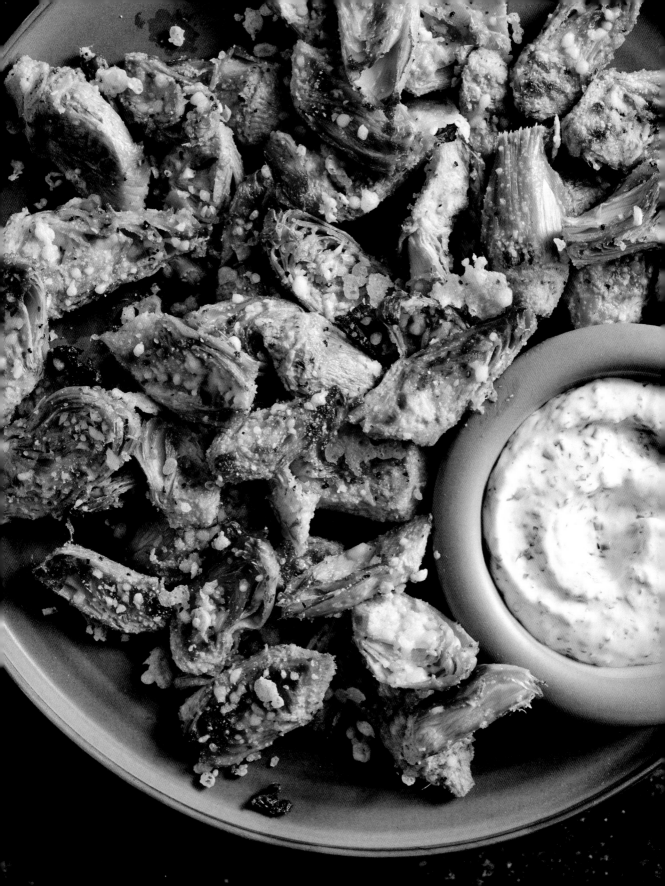

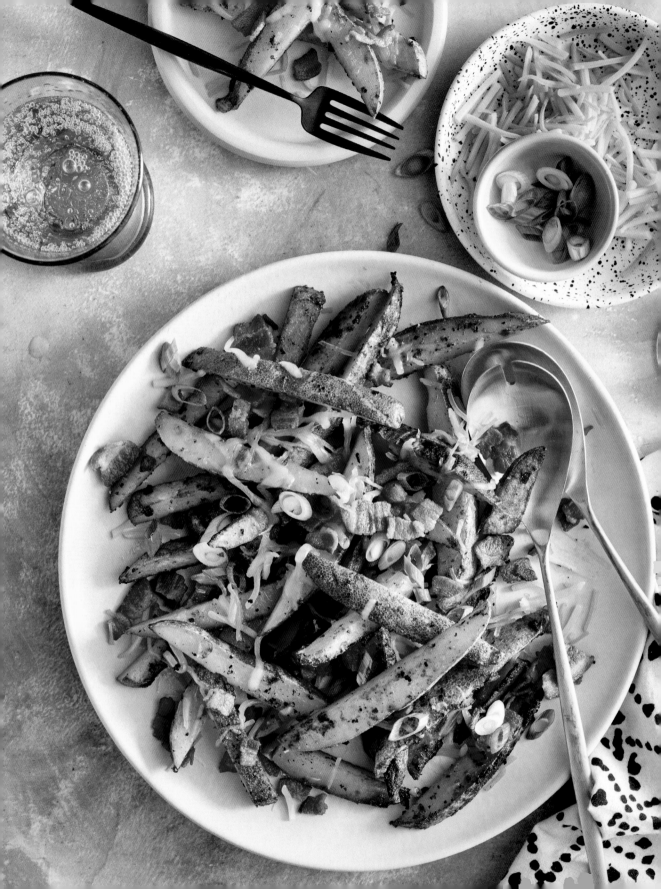

J's Loaded Potatoes

It's a special moment when one of your kids says, "Let me make dinner for everyone tonight." My oldest son, Jorden, is an amazing cook. On one of those special moments when he made family dinner, he came up with this spin on loaded fries using all organic ingredients.

Cut the potatoes into medium fries (½- to ¾-inch thick). Toss in a large bowl with the olive oil, salt, pepper, chili powder, garlic powder, and onion powder. Set aside.

Heat a large skillet or cast-iron pan over medium heat. Add the bacon and cook until crispy, about 5 minutes. Remove with a slotted spoon to a paper towel–lined plate.

Carefully pour out all but 2 tablespoons of the bacon fat from the pan. Add the onions to the pan and cook for about 3 minutes, until soft.

Add the butter and the potatoes, give them a stir, then cover with a lid. Cook for 15 minutes, stirring every 5 minutes. Remove the lid and cook for another 5 minutes, stirring occasionally until the potatoes are tender and crispy in places.

Spread the bacon pieces and cheese evenly on top and re-cover. Reduce the heat to low and cook for just a couple of minutes, until the cheese has melted. Serve and enjoy.

Serves 4 to 6

4 medium white potatoes, scrubbed but not peeled

3 tablespoons olive oil

1 teaspoon kosher salt

1 teaspoon black pepper

1 teaspoon chili powder

1 teaspoon garlic powder

1 teaspoon onion powder

4 slices bacon, diced

⅓ cup diced white onion (about ¼ small onion)

2 tablespoons unsalted grass-fed butter

¾ cup mixed shredded cheese (your choice)

Avocado Fries

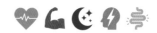

Whether it's game day, a holiday get-together, or a day you're hankering for something to dip (without all of the ancillary carbs of ordinary fries), this recipe is a winner!

Preheat the oven to 425°F. Line a baking sheet with parchment paper.

Bring out three shallow bowls. Pour the flour into one, crack the eggs into the second and whisk them to combine, and stir together the breadcrumbs, salt, pepper, paprika, garlic powder, and onion powder in the last one.

Cut the avocados in half and remove the pits. Cut each half in half, remove the skin, and slice each quarter into thirds. You should have 24 slices total.

Working with one slice at a time, dredge in the flour, followed by the eggs and then the breadcrumb mixture, to coat completely with each. Place on the baking sheet, not touching.

Coat the avocado slices with cooking spray. Bake for 8 minutes. Carefully flip the fries and coat with more cooking spray. Bake for another 8 to 10 minutes, until golden brown.

Let cool for a few minutes, then serve with ranch dressing.

Serves 4 to 6

½ cup gluten-free flour

1½ cups gluten-free panko breadcrumbs (we typically use Ian's)

2 large organic eggs

¾ teaspoon fine sea salt

¾ teaspoon black pepper

1½ teaspoons paprika

¾ teaspoon garlic powder

¾ teaspoon onion powder

2 firm ripe avocados

Coconut or olive oil cooking spray

Smarter Ranch Dressing (page 286)

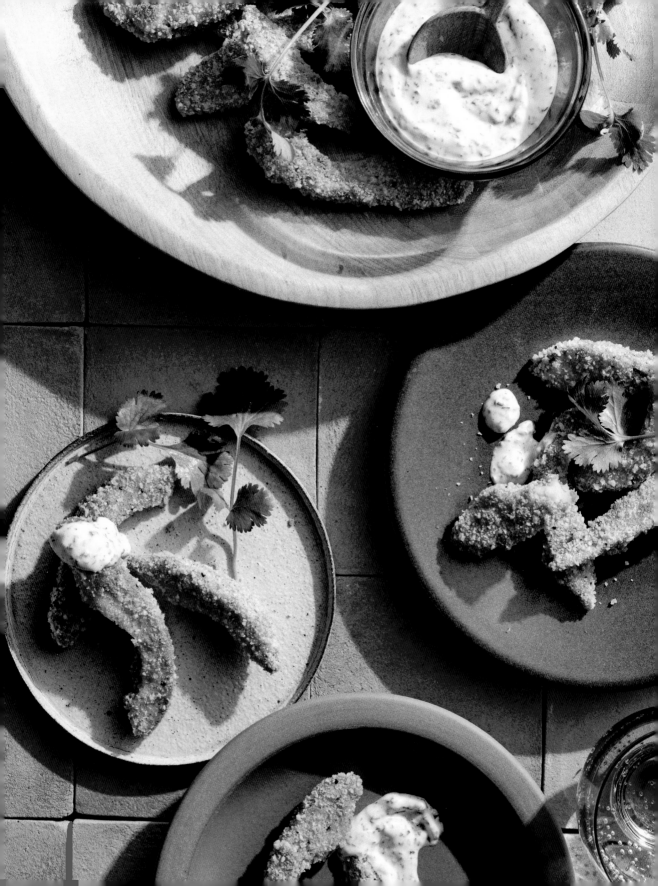

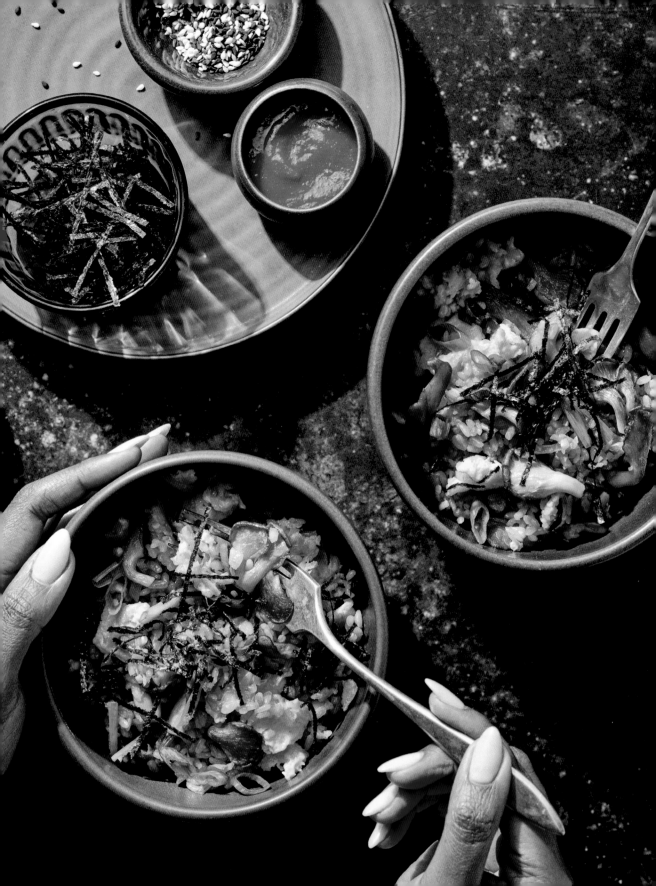

Mushroom Fried Rice

Not only does the upgraded cooking oil make this fried rice superior to what's served at most restaurants, the way that the rice itself is prepared dramatically increases its benefits to the microbiome and reduces its impact on blood sugar. By using rice that is cooked and then cooled (preferably even refrigerated), it significantly increases the resistant starch ratio of the rice. A study published in *The American Journal of Clinical Nutrition* found that resistant starch has profound effects on improving insulin sensitivity. Mushrooms are a great addition because they make this dish more hearty, but you can sub in any veggies you like—broccoli, zucchini, even frozen peas and carrots. It makes a great side dish for simply cooked chicken, steak, or fish, and it's also fitting as a vegetarian main course. And if you'd like to add a spicy kick, just drizzle on a bit of sriracha hot sauce.[13]

Cut the mushrooms away from their dirty base if they're still attached and tear into bite-sized pieces. Thinly slice the top third of the scallions (the greenest end) and set aside. Cut the remaining two-thirds in half lengthwise and then into 1-inch pieces.

Heat 2 tablespoons of the oil in a 10- or 12-inch safe nonstick sauté pan over medium-high heat. Add the mushrooms, season with salt, and cook for 3 to 5 minutes, until starting to brown. Add the scallion pieces, garlic, and ginger and cook for another 30 seconds.

Add the rice and cook for 2 more minutes, stirring every so often to make sure the rice isn't sticking. Make a well in the center, add the remaining tablespoon oil and crack in the eggs. Stir the eggs with a wooden spoon to scramble them until cooked through.

Mix the eggs into the rice mixture, then stir in sliced scallions and soy sauce. Transfer to a serving bowl. Garnish with nori and/or sriracha, if you like.

Serves 4

- **½ pound oyster mushrooms**
- **2 scallions**
- **3 tablespoons avocado oil**
- **Sea salt and black pepper**
- **2 garlic cloves, minced**
- **1-inch piece of ginger, minced**
- **2 cups cooked and cooled white or brown rice**
- **2 large organic eggs**
- **3 tablespoons soy sauce or nama shoyu (non-heat treated soy sauce)**
- **Thinly sliced nori or kelp flakes and sriracha hot sauce (optional)**

Easy Quinoa and Cauliflower "Pilaf"

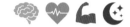

This combination of tasty, real-food plant fibers pairs great with Salisbury Steak Meatballs (page 218), Sheet Pan Fish with Mayo-Lemon Sauce and Asparagus (page 198), and Oven-Roasted Chicken Thighs with Olives (page 201). If you are cooking the quinoa yourself, using chicken broth will give it even more of that classic pilaf flavor.

Heat a 10- or 12-inch skillet over medium heat. Add 1 tablespoon of the butter and the olive oil. When the butter has melted, add the onion and a good pinch of salt and pepper. Sauté over medium-low heat for 3 to 5 minutes, until tender and translucent but not brown.

Add the cauliflower, turn the heat up to medium and cook for another 3 minutes, stirring often, until the cauliflower is just cooked through.

Add the quinoa and the remaining tablespoon butter. Cover, turn off the heat, and let the pilaf steam for 2 minutes. Give it a stir, taste for seasoning and adjust with salt and/or pepper, and serve.

Serves 4

2 tablespoons unsalted grass-fed butter

1 tablespoon olive oil

½ small yellow onion, minced

Sea salt and black pepper

1½ cups grated or riced cauliflower (about ½ small head)

1½ cups cooked quinoa

Better Brussels Sprouts

If there was a mascot for disliked vegetables, it would be the Brussels sprout. I get it. The problem is, this underappreciated vegetable is usually prepared in ways that don't complement its personality. I never thought I would like Brussels sprouts until my wife made these. Now we absolutely love them and look forward to their performance on nutritional game days.

Position two racks in the upper and lower thirds of the oven. Preheat the oven to 425°F.

Toss together the Brussels sprouts, lemon slices, olive oil, garlic, bacon, thyme, salt, and pepper in a large bowl. Transfer to a large rimmed baking sheet and spread in an even layer.

Roast on the upper rack without stirring for 10 minutes. Switch to the lower rack and continue roasting, without stirring, until the sprouts are lightly browned and tender, 8 to 10 minutes longer. Transfer to a serving dish. Sprinkle with the parm, if using.

Serves 4

- **1 pound Brussels sprouts, trimmed and halved, or quartered if large**
- **½ small lemon, sliced**
- **2 tablespoons olive oil**
- **1 tablespoon garlic powder or 2 garlic cloves, sliced**
- **3 slices bacon, diced**
- **1½ teaspoons dried thyme**
- **½ teaspoon fine sea salt**
- **¼ teaspoon black pepper**
- **3 tablespoons finely shredded parmesan cheese (optional)**

Kelp Noodles
with Pesto

These noodles are made from nutrient-rich sea veggies and are completely gluten-free. You can find them online or in the refrigerated section at many health food stores. You can serve this alongside a variety of dishes, like the Honey Sriracha Salmon, page 193! Or you can even add some leftover veggies and a simple protein to make it a complete meal.

Rinse the noodles in a colander under cold water, then transfer them to a large bowl. Cover with hot tap water and mix in the lemon juice and baking soda. Let the noodles sit for 5 minutes to soften. Drain, then transfer to a serving bowl.

Toss with the pesto, season to taste with salt and pepper, and serve.

Serves 4

1 (12-ounce) packet kelp noodles

Juice of 1 lemon

2 teaspoons baking soda

3 tablespoons Superfood Pesto (page 284) or your favorite store-bought pesto

Sea salt and black pepper

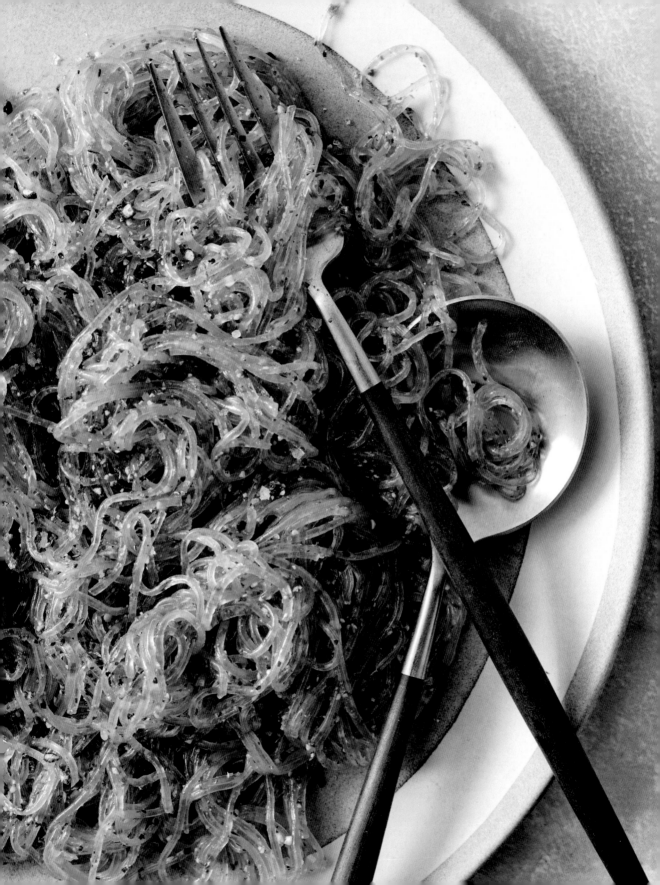

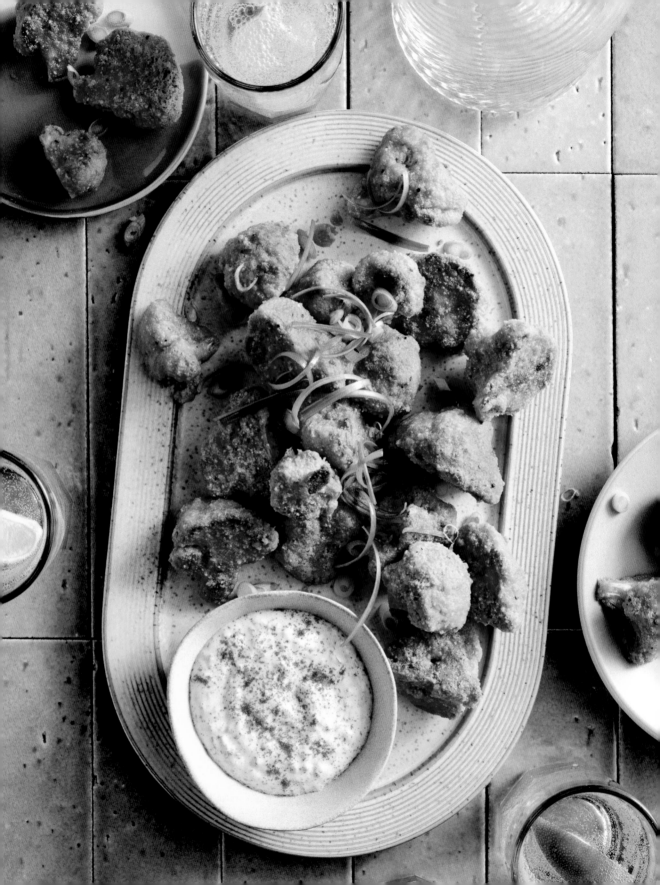

Buffalo Cauliflower

Before Ricky Bobby and Cal Naughton, Jr. performed shake'n bake on the NASCAR track in the movie *Talladega Nights*, shake'n bake was being performed in kitchens all over the country thanks to the premade coating being marketed to families. The goal of shake'n bake was to get your dish crispy without frying. That's exactly what this recipe brings to the table. It's an awesome appetizer, great for when you have company over. I highly recommend using the Smarter Ranch Dressing for dipping!

Preheat the oven to 425°F. Line a baking sheet with parchment paper.

In a large resealable bag or bowl with a lid (it should be large enough to hold all of the cauliflower), combine the almond flour, cornstarch, garlic powder, turmeric, pepper, and salt.

Whisk the egg and milk in a large bowl and add the cauliflower. Mix until all of the florets are fully coated.

Add the cauliflower to the almond flour coating. Seal the bag or cover the bowl and shake to coat the cauliflower.

Brush or spray the parchment with avocado oil and arrange the cauliflower in a single layer on the baking sheet. Drizzle or spray more avocado oil over the top. Roast in the oven for 25 minutes or until browned and tender.

While the cauliflower is in the oven, melt the butter in a microwave-safe bowl or small saucepan. Whisk in the hot sauce.

Pour the buffalo sauce over the cauliflower and carefully mix on the baking sheet to try and coat most of the pieces. Push the cauliflower and sauce towards the center of the baking sheet and broil for about 3 minutes, until the sauce is bubbling and starting to brown on top.

Scatter over the sliced scallion. Serve with ranch dressing on the side, if you like!

Serves 4

1 cup almond flour

3 tablespoons cornstarch

1 teaspoon garlic powder

1 teaspoon ground turmeric

½ teaspoon black pepper

½ teaspoon fine sea salt

1 large organic egg

2 tablespoons unsweetened almond milk or other milk of your choice

1 medium head cauliflower, cut into 1- to 2-inch florets

About 2 tablespoons avocado oil or avocado oil spray

4 tablespoons unsalted grass-fed butter

¼ cup Frank's RedHot sauce

1 scallion, thinly sliced

½ cup Smarter Ranch Dressing (page 286; optional)

Grilled Zucchini & Peppers with Italian Herbs

In Chapter Three we noted how foods in the gourd family, like zucchini, have been found to support microbiome diversity and blood sugar regulation. This recipe is an amazing way to make zucchini and just about any other veggies on the grill. Asparagus, onions, or eggplant would also be great, for example.

Heat the grill to medium-high.

Remove the ends from the zucchini. Cut the zucchini lengthwise into roughly ½-inch-thick slices. Remove the stems, cores, and seeds from the bell peppers and cut each pepper into three pieces. Toss the veggies with about 3 tablespoons olive oil and season generously with salt and pepper.

Whisk together 2 tablespoons olive oil with the vinegar, Italian seasoning, garlic, and chili flakes (if using). Season the dressing to taste with salt and pepper and set aside.

Arrange the veggies in a single layer on the grill and cook, turning once, for about 3 minutes per side, until nicely charred and tender.

Remove to a serving platter and pour over the dressing (see Note). Serve hot or at room temperature.

Note: By pouring over the flavorful marinade *after* the veggies are cooked instead of before, the flavors have a chance to really soak into the hot veggies.

Serves 4

3 medium zucchini

2 red bell peppers

Olive oil

Sea salt and black pepper

2 tablespoons apple cider vinegar

1 teaspoon Italian seasoning

1 small garlic clove, minced

¼ teaspoon chili flakes (optional)

Brain-Boosting Garlicky Spinach

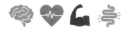

As we covered earlier, scientists at Chicago's Rush University Medical Center found that people who ate one to two servings of leafy green vegetables like spinach each day experienced fewer memory problems and less cognitive decline. I can't stress enough how extraordinary this is. It's so simple, but we have to make it a *must* to actually do it. This spinach recipe takes the brain benefits up a few more notches with the healthy helping of fresh garlic. It's fast, easy to make, and it will help keep cognitive decline—and maybe even vampires—away.

Heat the oil in a large pot or Dutch oven over medium heat. Add the garlic and sauté for 20 to 30 seconds, until fragrant but still white. Add all the spinach, the onion powder, salt, and pepper to the pot; toss with the garlic and oil. Cook, stirring often, until the spinach is just wilted, 3 to 5 minutes. Serve immediately.

Serves 2 to 4

2 tablespoons extra virgin olive oil

1 tablespoon minced garlic (2 to 3 cloves)

1 pound baby spinach

½ teaspoon onion powder

1 teaspoon fine sea salt

1 teaspoon black pepper

Snacks

CHAPTER TEN Sharing and eating tasty snacks can instantly bring folks together. These nostalgic snacks, made with smarter ingredients, are a perfect match for making memories that last forever.

Speedy Superfood Guacamole

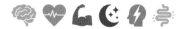

There isn't another guacamole recipe that comes close to the simplicity and nutrient density of this one. It is one of my go-to snacks and toppings—and the secret ingredient in the recipe takes the green to another level!

In a large bowl, mash up the avocados with a fork until smooth. Add the salsa, spirulina, cayenne, lemon juice, and salt to taste. Mix well. Serve immediately or cover and chill in the refrigerator before serving.

Serves 4

3 ripe avocados, pitted and peeled

⅓ cup salsa (your choice; we typically use a medium-hot salsa)

1 teaspoon spirulina powder

¼ teaspoon cayenne pepper

2 teaspoons fresh lemon juice

Sea salt

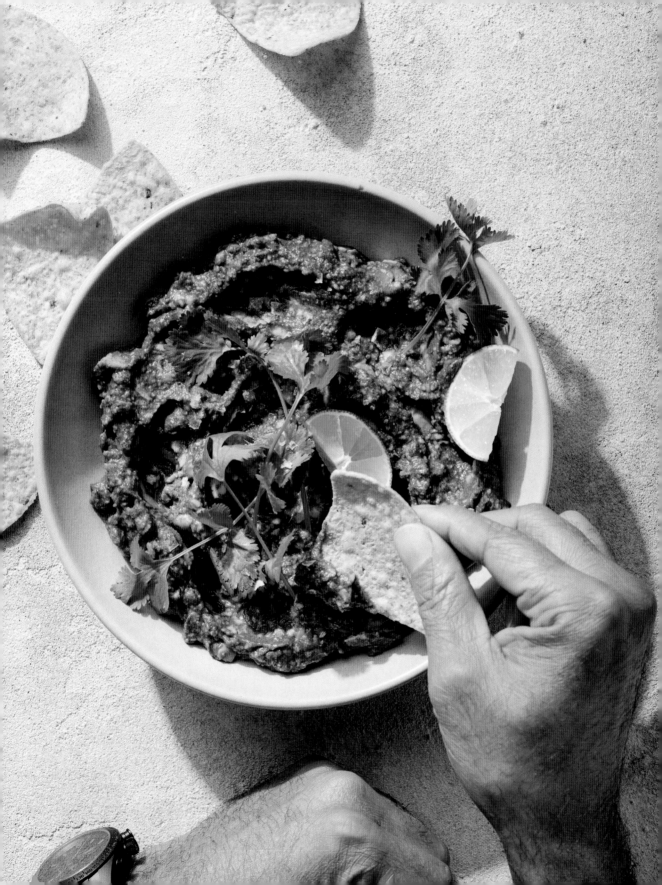

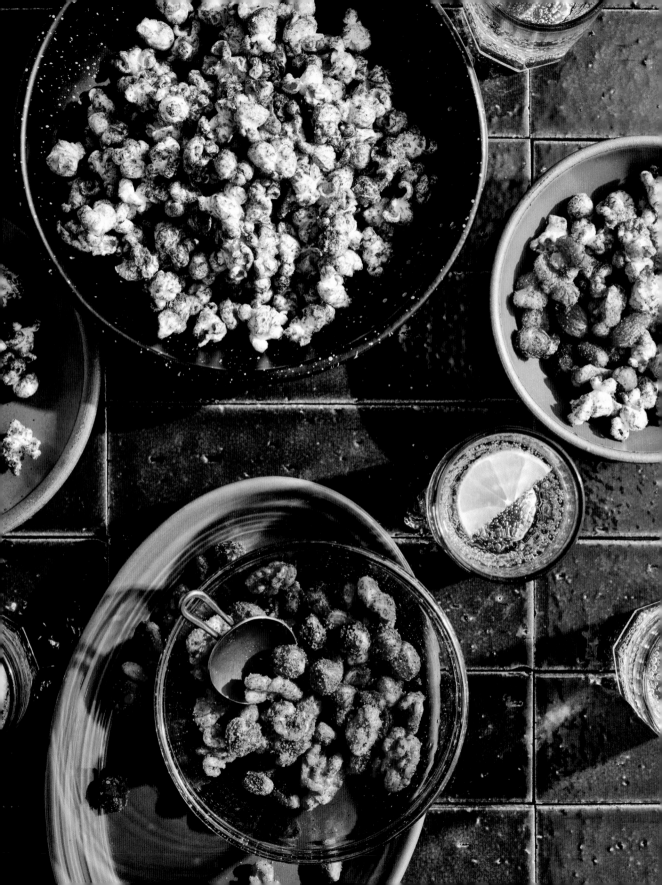

Smoky Spicy Mixed Nuts

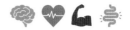

Roasted nuts can be an amazing snack that supports your brain, heart, and microbiome. But the low-quality oils used in prepackaged roasted nuts can take a good thing and sabotage it. This incredible recipe combines some of the healthiest nuts *plus* a health-supportive oil to make a snack worthy of your taste buds. These are perfect as a snack on their own, but they're also great added to salads or grain bowls.

Preheat the oven to 350°F.

Toss the nuts with 1 teaspoon of the avocado oil and the apple cider vinegar. Transfer to a baking sheet. Roast for 5 to 10 minutes, until the nuts are toasted but not burned. (Be sure to watch them closely!)

While the nuts cook, combine the garlic powder, turmeric, paprika, cayenne, ground chipotle, nutritional yeast, ¼ teaspoon salt, ⅛ teaspoon pepper, and the coconut sugar in a medium bowl.

Transfer the hot nuts to the spice mixture and toss to combine. Add the remaining teaspoon avocado oil, give it another toss, and season to taste with more salt and pepper.

Eat warm, or let cool and store in an airtight container at room temperature for up to a week.

Serves 4

- **1 cup assorted raw nuts (a mix of almonds, walnuts, pistachios and hazelnuts is nice)**
- **2 teaspoons avocado oil**
- **2 teaspoons apple cider vinegar**
- **½ teaspoon garlic powder**
- **¼ teaspoon ground turmeric**
- **½ teaspoon paprika**
- **⅛ teaspoon cayenne pepper**
- **¼ teaspoon ground chipotle**
- **1 teaspoon nutritional yeast**
- **Kosher salt and black pepper**
- **½ teaspoon coconut sugar**

Marinated Olives

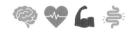

This simple recipe can amp up the taste and health benefits of olives tenfold. They're great as an antioxidant-rich snack or a flavorful addition to your meals.

Use a vegetable peeler to remove all the zest from the lemon in large strips. (Remove only the colored outside; try and leave out any white pith.) Put the zest in a large jar (one that will hold all of the olives). Squeeze in the lemon juice. Add the olives, thyme, and oregano.

Heat the olive oil, garlic, and chili flakes in a saucepan over medium heat to a low simmer. Carefully pour the oil mixture over the olives. Let cool to room temperature. Cover and refrigerate for at least 24 hours before serving.

Serves 6 to 8

1 lemon

1½ cups mixed olives (with pits)

½ teaspoon dried thyme

½ teaspoon dried oregano

⅔ cup olive oil

4 garlic cloves, peeled and smashed

½ teaspoon chili flakes

Jicama with Chipotle Salt and Lime

Carrot and celery sticks are cool, but there's a new snackable raw veggie in town. Jicama has been enjoyed for thousands of years and prized for its variety of nutrients. Today it's having a resurgence in popular culture, most notably for its prebiotic benefits. This recipe is easy to make and a great veggie to prepare in advance because it doesn't oxidize quickly and turn brown as it sits.

Make the chili salt by mixing the salt, ground chipotle, and chili powder in a small bowl. Squeeze the lime juice over the jicama sticks and sprinkle each with a little chili salt just before eating.

Serves 4

1 teaspoon kosher salt

½ teaspoon ground chipotle

¼ teaspoon chili powder

Juice of 2 limes

1 medium jicama, peeled and cut into sticks

Quick and Easy Deviled Eggs

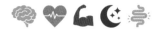

Enjoy these micronutrient-packed deviled eggs without all the heavy lifting. It's a cheat code on deviled eggs that delivers familiar flavors and satisfaction, but none of the usual mixing and mashing required.

Place the eggs in a medium pot and add enough cold water to completely cover the eggs—plus about an inch or so additional. Place the pot over high heat and bring to a rolling boil. Cover the pot and remove from the heat. Set a timer for 8 minutes.

Fill a large bowl with water and ice. Once the 8 minutes are up, remove the eggs and place them in the ice bath until cool, then carefully peel.

Cut the eggs in half lengthwise. Top each half with about 1½ teaspoons of the miso mayo and the kimchi (if using). Sprinkle over kelp flakes and enjoy!

Serves 4

4 large organic eggs

2 tablespoons Miso Mayo (page 281)

2 tablespoons chopped kimchi (optional)

Kelp flakes or thinly sliced toasted nori

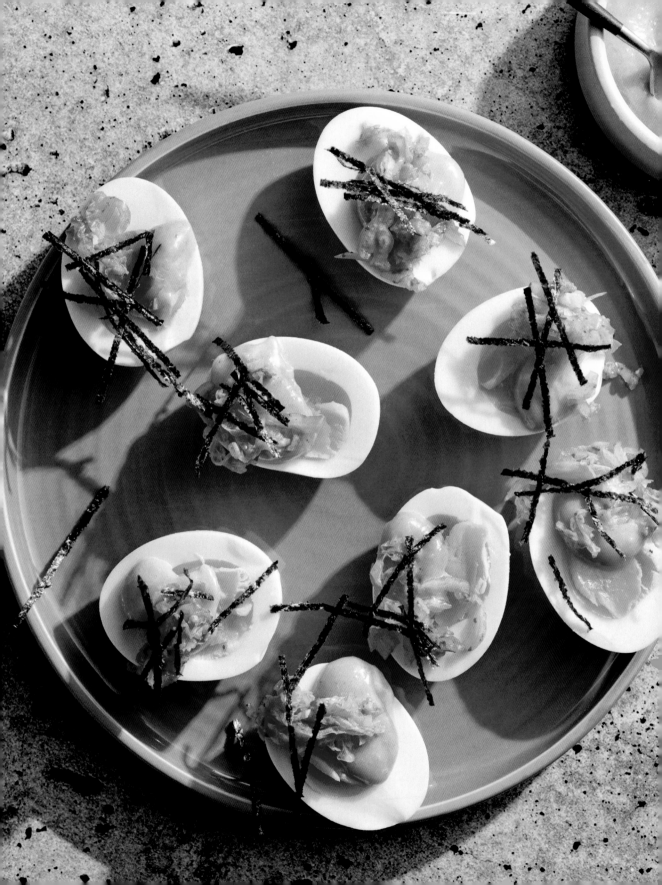

Arugula Hummus

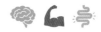

A study published in the *Journal of the American Dietetic Association* found that test subjects consuming about 3 ounces of chickpeas per day had reduced levels of insulin resistance. Chickpeas are the star ingredient in the gloried "dip" called hummus. I put dip in quotes because I've seen people dig hummus out of a container with pita bread, veggie slices, their fingers, and even a pen cap one time. (People who love hummus tend to love it in a social misconduct kind of way.) But the chickpeas themselves (also called garbanzo beans), when prepared properly to reduce the potential lectins and antinutrients, are a viable source of protein with a slightly higher ratio of fat and less carbs than some other beans. Look for Eden brand chickpeas if you can find them (they're pressure cooked which helps reduce potential antinutrients). Serve with your favorite cut-up veggies for dipping![14]

Place the chickpeas, arugula, garlic, lemon juice, cumin, olive oil, and tahini in a blender or food processor and blitz until smooth, adding water as needed, 1 tablespoon at a time, until you get a nice, creamy consistency. Season to taste with salt and pepper.

Note: You could easily make this spinach hummus instead of arugula. Also, finding the right balance of flavors is all about personal taste, so adjust with more lemon, cumin, or grated garlic to suit your desires!

Serves 4 to 6

1 (15-ounce) can chickpeas, rinsed and drained

1 cup packed baby arugula (see Note)

1 garlic clove, sliced

Juice of 1 lemon

½ teaspoon ground cumin

3 tablespoons olive oil

2 tablespoons tahini

Sea salt and black pepper

E. T. Popcorn

This is an awesome movie snack! My kids enjoy the "alien" green color. Plus, this cosmic snack actually delivers some bona fide nutrition along with the popcorn kernels.

Heat 1 tablespoon of the avocado oil and 3 popcorn kernels in a covered 4-quart saucepan or Dutch oven over medium heat. When you hear the corn kernels pop, add the remaining popcorn. Continue cooking, shaking the pan every 30 seconds or so with the lid ajar, until the popping slows to 1 to 2 seconds between pops.

While the popcorn pops, combine the nutritional yeast, onion powder, garlic powder, spirulina, cayenne, and salt in a small bowl.

Transfer the popped popcorn to a large bowl and toss with the remaining 2 tablespoons avocado oil, making sure the oil coats all the popcorn. Sprinkle over the spice mixture, toss to coat all the kernels. Enjoy!

Makes about 4 cups; serves 2 to 4

3 tablespoons avocado oil

¼ cup popcorn kernels

2 tablespoons nutritional yeast

½ teaspoon onion powder

½ teaspoon garlic powder

1 teaspoon spirulina powder

⅛ teaspoon cayenne pepper, or to taste

½ teaspoon kosher salt, or more to taste

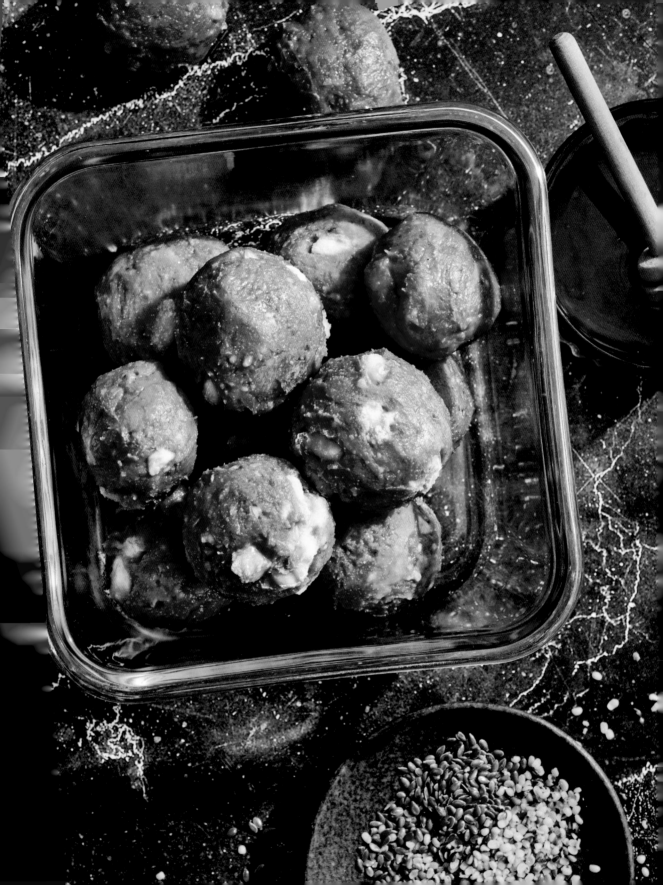

Cashew Butter Planets

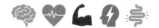

These little treats are out of this world. When you're orbiting your kitchen in search of a frozen treat, you'll find that these Cashew Butter Planets will make your taste buds lift off while providing an array of micronutrients. This recipe has bonbon vibes, but it's far more nutritious. Plus, you can add so many ingredients you love into the mix. Some great options include cacao nibs, coconut butter, and/or bee pollen.

Place the flaxseeds in a small bowl or ramekin and mix in the water. Set aside for at least 1 hour to make a gel (see Note).

Transfer the gel to a large bowl and stir in the banana, nut butter, hemp seeds, honey, and salt. Mix well.

Line a lidded freezer-safe container with parchment paper.

Grab enough of the mixture to make a golf ball–sized sphere and roll between your hands. (It doesn't have to be a perfect ball at all!) Place in the container. Repeat to make 15 to 20 balls, making sure that you don't place them too close together. If your container isn't that big, place a sheet of parchment on top of the first layer of cashew planets, then add a second layer.

Put a tight-fitting lid on the container and place in the freezer for at least 4 hours. Take a Cashew Butter Planet out of the freezer as desired and enjoy!

Note: Make sure to soak the flaxseeds for at least 1 hour so you have a nice gel to bind these treats together.

Makes 15 to 20 planets

1 tablespoon whole flaxseeds

2 tablespoons water

1 ripe banana, diced

2 cups cashew butter

2 tablespoons hulled hemp seeds

2 tablespoons raw honey

¼ teaspoon fine sea salt

Smarter Granola Bars

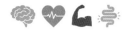

These real-food bars blow conventional prepackaged bars out of the water! High-quality protein, a variety of micronutrients—and a hint of sweetness brings it all together.

Line an 8 by 8-inch baking dish with parchment paper.

Toast the almonds, hazelnuts, and coconut flakes in a dry sauté pan over medium heat, stirring occasionally, for 3 to 5 minutes, until the coconut is just starting to brown.

Transfer to a bowl along with the cereal, flaxseeds, hemp seeds, and kosher salt.

Heat the honey, nut butter, and coconut oil in the same sauté pan over medium heat until warm and melted.

Pour over the nut mixture and stir to combine. Transfer to the baking dish and press into the pan evenly. Sprinkle with sea salt, if using. Let cool to room temperature.

Cover and transfer to the refrigerator to firm up for at least 30 minutes before cutting into bars. Store the bars in the fridge, covered, for up to 5 days.

Makes 12 bars

½ cup raw almonds, roughly chopped

½ cup raw hazelnuts, roughly chopped

½ cup unsweetened coconut flakes

1 cup puffed millet or puffed rice cereal

2 tablespoons ground flaxseeds

¼ cup hulled hemp seeds

¼ teaspoon kosher salt

⅓ cup raw honey

⅓ cup salted, unsweetened almond butter or other nut butter

1 tablespoon coconut oil

Flaky sea salt (optional)

Pumpkin Muffins

There are two things you need to know about this incredible gluten-free muffin recipe: 1) these muffins taste amazing! and 2) the unique combination of ingredients helps lower the glycemic load you'd get from typical muffins. If you'd like an extra wow-factor, while they're still warm add a tiny bit of grass-fed butter on top right before you serve them.

Preheat the oven to 350°F. Line a muffin tray with 12 paper liners.

Whisk together the almond flour, cassava flour, cinnamon, nutmeg, cloves, salt, baking powder, and baking soda in a medium mixing bowl.

In a large mixing bowl, whisk together the sugar and pumpkin. Crack in the eggs one at a time, whisking after each addition. Whisk in the avocado oil.

Pour the dry ingredients into the wet ingredients and use a spatula to gently mix everything together.

Divide the batter between the 12 muffin cups and garnish each with a sprinkle of pumpkin seeds, if using. Transfer to the oven and bake for 20 to 25 minutes, until a toothpick inserted into the center comes out clean. Let cool before serving.

Makes 12 muffins

1 cup almond flour

1 cup cassava flour

2 teaspoons ground cinnamon

½ teaspoon ground nutmeg

⅛ teaspoon ground cloves

½ teaspoon kosher salt

1 teaspoon baking powder

½ teaspoon baking soda

¾ cup coconut sugar

¾ cup canned pumpkin

3 large organic eggs

½ cup avocado oil

2 tablespoons pumpkin seeds (optional)

Desserts

CHAPTER ELEVEN   In this section, classic treats like ice cream, slushies, and chocolate bars are getting a nutritional makeover to make you feel better than ever. The flavor experiences are out of this world, but the nutrition is grounded with real, health-enhancing foods.

Superfood Chocolate Bark

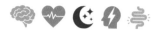

You'll never have to reach for a processed candy bar again. Keep a stash of this in the freezer for anytime you're craving something sweet. It's also a delectable, easy dessert or snack to share with guests. This chocolatey bark is customizable as well—you can sprinkle any mix of nuts, seeds, and superfoods you like on top!

Line a 9 by 12-inch baking sheet or 8 by 8-inch baking pan with parchment paper.

Heat the coconut oil in a small saucepan over medium-low heat until melted, then turn off the heat. Whisk in the cacao and honey until thoroughly mixed.

Spread the mixture onto the baking sheet. Top evenly with the hazelnuts, hemp seeds, cacao nibs, goji berries, and the salt, if using.

Put the baking sheet in the freezer for 15 to 20 minutes to firm up. Break into pieces and store in the fridge or freezer in a tightly covered container.

Serves 4

½ cup coconut oil

⅔ cup raw cacao powder

¼ cup raw honey

½ cup hazelnuts, toasted

1 tablespoon hulled hemp seeds

1 tablespoon cacao nibs

1 tablespoon dried goji berries

2 teaspoons flaky sea salt (optional)

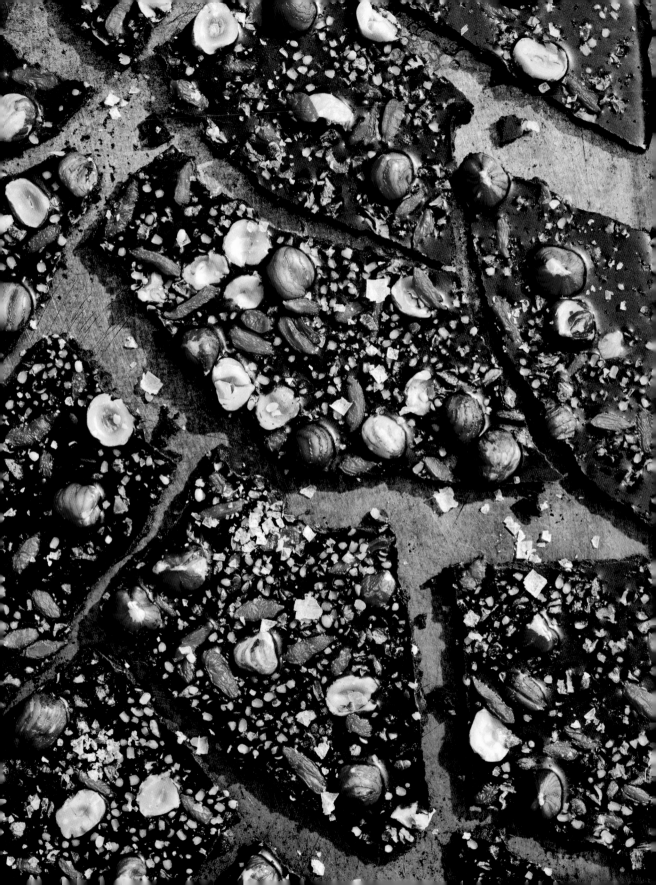

Smarter Snickers Bites

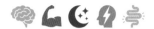

These have all the crunchy, peanut-y, caramel-y taste of a candy bar with none of the ultra-processed ingredients. Plus, not only do these ingredients taste amazing, they're clinically proven to support brain health, cardiovascular health, and more.

Place the peanut butter, honey, coconut oil, dates, vanilla extract, and kosher salt in a high-speed blender or food processor and blend until the mixture clumps up and forms a sort of ball, about 1 minute. (Don't worry if the oils separate a bit.) Transfer to a small bowl and stir in peanuts and hemp seeds. Cover and transfer to the fridge for at least 30 minutes to firm up.

While the filling chills, make the chocolate coating. Heat the coconut oil over medium-low heat in a small saucepan until melted. Turn off the heat and whisk in the cacao and honey. Transfer to a bowl and set aside for about 10 minutes to cool and thicken.

Line a 9 by 12-inch baking sheet or 8 by 8-inch baking dish with parchment paper.

Roll the filling into 20 little balls. (Again, don't worry if the oils separate a bit and the mixture feels "greasy"; it will firm up in the freezer.) Using a fork, roll the balls in the chocolate coating, then transfer to the baking sheet. Sprinkle each with a pinch of flaky salt and put in the freezer for at least 1 hour to set up. Take out the desired amount of Smarter Snickers Bites to enjoy (allow them to unthaw for a few minutes if you'd like them a bit softer) and leave the rest stored in the freezer for later snacking.

Makes 20 bites

FILLING

½ cup salted, unsweetened peanut butter

¼ cup raw honey

3 tablespoons coconut oil, melted and cooled slightly

4 Medjool dates, pitted and roughly chopped

1 teaspoon vanilla extract

¼ teaspoon kosher salt

¼ cup raw peanuts, roasted, cooled, and roughly chopped

¼ cup hulled hemp seeds

CHOCOLATE COATING

¼ cup coconut oil

⅓ cup raw cacao or cocoa powder

2 tablespoons raw honey

TO FINISH

Flaky sea salt

No-Churn Hazelnut Chocolate Ice Cream

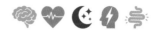

This is the easiest ice cream you will ever make! And such a crowd-pleaser. With the chocolate-hazelnut combo, it has a Nutella vibe to it—so creamy and satisfying. Home ice cream makers are great devices if you get a good one, but they're not necessary if you have some ingenuity and some delicious ingredients. Plus, you have ultimate quality control and can add any fun toppings you like when serving.

Preheat the oven to 350°F.

Put the hazelnuts in a baking dish and toast in the oven for about 5 minutes, until golden. Let cool slightly, then rub off the skins with a clean dish towel. Roughly chop the hazelnuts. Set aside.

Combine the cream, condensed milk, vanilla extract, salt, and cacao in the bowl of a stand mixer fitted with the whisk attachment. (You can also use a large bowl and an electric hand mixer.) Whisk on medium-high speed until the mixture holds stiff peaks, about 3 minutes.

Transfer the mixture to a 9-inch loaf pan or 8 by 8-inch baking pan. Top with the chopped hazelnuts and the cacao nibs, if using.

Cover with plastic wrap and place in the freezer for at least 4 hours to firm up. Serve or keep it stored in the freezer for later use.

Serves 6 to 8

½ cup raw hazelnuts

2 cups grass-fed heavy cream

1 (14-ounce) can sweetened condensed milk

1 teaspoon vanilla extract

Pinch of fine sea salt

3 tablespoons raw cacao or cocoa powder, sifted

2 tablespoons cacao nibs (optional)

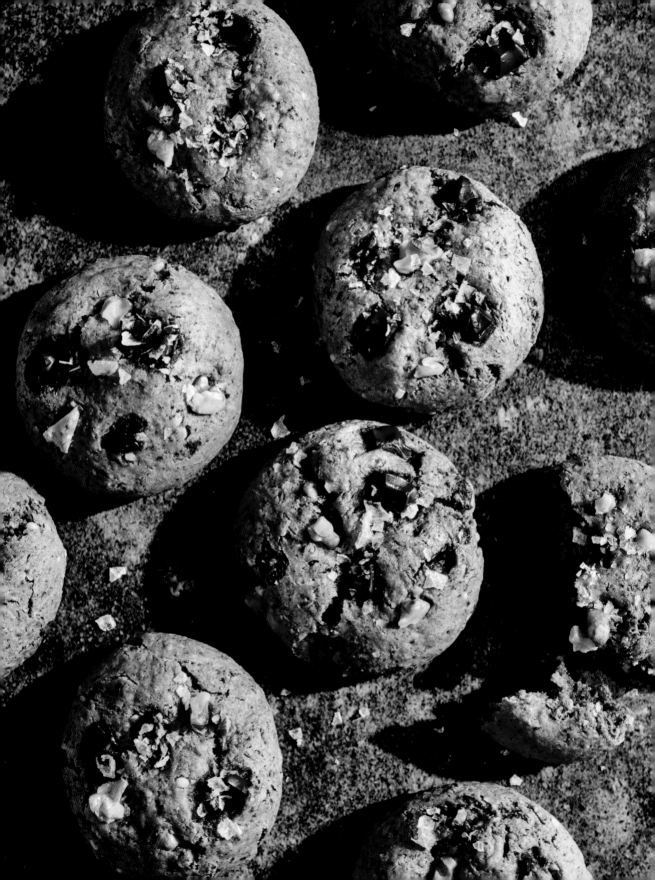

Almond Butter Chocolate Chip Cookies

A lot of healthier cookie recipes mean well by trying to finagle in a bunch of nonglycemic sweeteners (even though they're still highly processed), and try to convince us that the cookie tastes good. In reality, their cookies taste like Pepto-Bismol, but without the soothing aftereffects. If you're going to make a cookie, make a cookie! We can upgrade the quality immensely by using more whole, real-food ingredients. Plus we can skip on a lot of the additives and pesticides that are, without a doubt, littered within conventional cookies on the store shelves. This cookie recipe is a happy medium—a bridge between a scrumptious snack, real food, and healthy upgrades.

Preheat the oven to 375°F. Line a baking sheet with parchment paper.

Whisk together the sugar and baking soda. Stir in the almond butter and mix to combine. Crack in the egg. Mix in the chocolate chips, hemp seeds, flaxseeds, and walnuts.

Roll into 10 equal balls about the size of a golf ball and arrange evenly on the baking sheet. Gently press them down a bit with your fingers. Transfer to the oven and bake for 10 to 12 minutes, turning the pan front to back halfway through, until lightly golden.

Remove from the oven and sprinkle with flaky salt. Let cool to room temperature before eating.

Makes 10 cookies

- ⅓ cup coconut sugar
- ½ teaspoon baking soda
- ½ cup salted, unsweetened almond butter
- 1 large organic egg
- ¼ cup chocolate chips
- 2 tablespoons hulled hemp seeds
- ¼ cup ground flaxseeds
- ¼ cup walnuts, toasted and chopped
- Flaky sea salt

Cinnamon Bread Pudding with Caramel Sauce

There's no way I could make a family cookbook without including my wife's favorite dessert. On many of our date nights while living in St. Louis, Missouri, we'd go to our favorite restaurant for fun, quality time, and her favorite bread pudding. After moving to Los Angeles, we simply couldn't find a bread pudding that compared. That's when we decided to make one ourselves! This recipe is pure indulgence...but, of course, we found a way to make it using the best ingredients possible. Not even our favorite restaurant used all organic ingredients like we did, and I encourage you to do the same. Serve it warm with a scoop of vanilla ice cream if you like, but it's equally delicious with just the caramel sauce on top.

Preheat the oven to 350°F. Grease four 4-ounce ramekins generously with butter and place them on a baking sheet.

Whisk together the egg, egg yolk, milk, cream, sugar, salt, vanilla extract, and ground cinnamon in a large bowl. Mix in the bread and let soak for 10 minutes.

Divide the mixture between the ramekins, top each with ½ tablespoon of butter, and bake for 18 to 20 minutes, until puffed and lightly golden.

Meanwhile, make the sauce: Combine the butter, sugar, and cream in a small, heavy-bottomed saucepan. Bring the mixture up to a gentle simmer and cook, stirring constantly, for 2 minutes or until the sugar is melted and the sauce is slightly thickened. Set aside to keep warm.

Remove the puddings from the oven and let cool for 5 minutes.

Carefully run a butter knife around the edges and underneath, releasing the puddings from the ramekins. Using a dish towel to protect your hands, invert them onto serving plates. Spoon over the caramel sauce. Top each with a scoop of vanilla ice cream, if using.

Serves 4

BREAD PUDDING

2 tablespoons salted grass-fed butter, plus extra for the ramekins

1 large organic egg

1 large organic egg yolk

¾ cup grass-fed whole milk

¼ cup grass-fed heavy cream

2 tablespoons coconut sugar

Pinch of fine sea salt

½ teaspoon vanilla extract

½ teaspoon ground cinnamon

4 (1-inch-thick) slices brioche bread, cut into 1-inch cubes (about 4 cups total; see Note)

CARAMEL SAUCE

4 tablespoons unsalted grass-fed butter

¼ cup coconut sugar

¼ cup grass-fed heavy cream

TO SERVE

4 scoops vanilla ice cream (optional)

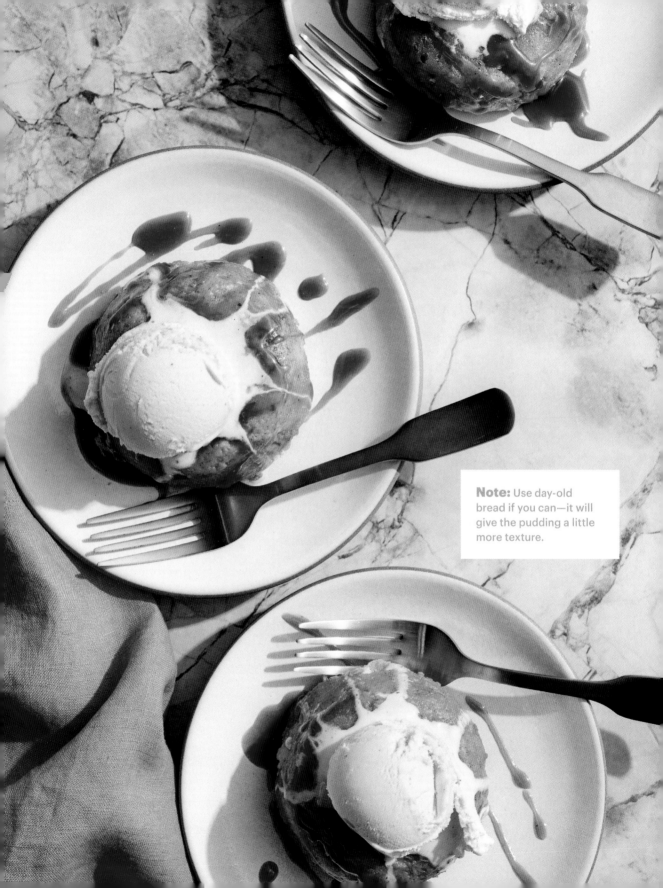

Note: Use day-old bread if you can—it will give the pudding a little more texture.

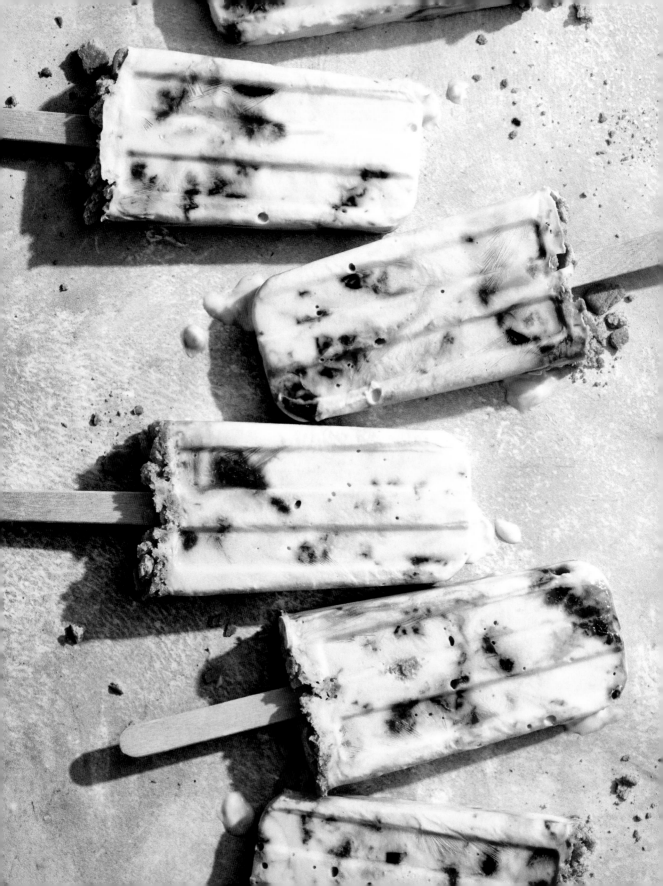

Cherry Frozen Yogurt Pops

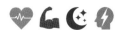

These yogurt pops are delicious enough to eat for dessert, but healthy enough to have for any occasion! Kids absolutely love them and they're fun to make together as a family.

Combine the cherries, 2 teaspoons of the honey, and the water in a small saucepan. Bring the mixture up to a simmer, then cook gently for about 5 minutes, until the cherries are warm and softened. Using a potato masher, crush the cherries, breaking them into small pieces. Set aside to cool for at least 5 minutes.

In a large bowl, whisk together the yogurt, the remaining 2 tablespoons honey, and the vanilla extract. Fold in the cherries, being careful not to overmix so you get some nice swirls.

Pour the mixture into 8 popsicle molds and sprinkle over the graham cracker crumbs. Add popsicle sticks, transfer to the freezer, and let sit for at least 4 hours to firm up. Serve or keep them stored in the freezer for later enjoyment.

Note: You could use any berry you like in place of the cherries, but you might need to adjust the amount of honey you use.

Serves 8

2 cups frozen pitted cherries (see Note)

2 teaspoons plus 2 tablespoons raw honey

1 tablespoon water

2 cups grass-fed whole milk Greek yogurt

½ teaspoon vanilla extract

¾ cup graham cracker crumbs

Lemonade Slushie

In Italy they would call this a granita, but at my house we call these lemonade slushies! They remind me of being a kid getting a snow cone or Slurpee, but this version is made without any of the high fructose corn syrup. As always, go for organic options with your ingredients (including sweeteners) whenever possible. This recipe does have a bit of cane sugar, but you can scale it up or down depending on the flavor you like—this is meant to be a sweet treat to have in your superhero utility belt when the occasion calls for it. We prefer our slushies a bit on the tart side (nice and refreshing on a hot day!) but feel free to add more honey and/or sugar to taste.

Bring a small saucepan of water up to a boil. Whisk together the lemon juice, sugar, and honey in an 8 by 8-inch metal baking pan. Pour in 1 cup of just-boiled water and whisk until the sugar and honey have dissolved. Stir in the cold water. Let the mixture cool to room temp.

Cover and place in the freezer for 2 hours. Remove the slushie from the freezer and use a fork to scrape up any frozen bits (especially around the edges), then return to the freezer for another hour. Remove, scrape with a fork, breaking up any new ice crystals, then return to the freezer for 1 more hour. Do one final scrape before serving. Or re-cover and leave in the freezer for up to 5 days.

Serves 4 to 6

¾ cup fresh lemon juice (about 4 to 5 lemons)

2 tablespoons organic cane sugar

2 tablespoons raw honey

1 cup cold water

Sweet Potato Chocolate Pudding

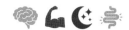

This rich, satisfying dessert can be as simple or as decadent as you want to make it. You can serve it with assorted berries, but it would also be a feast for the eyes with a little whipped cream and shaved chocolate on top. If you have a high-speed blender, it's worth using it here to get that super luscious texture, but a food processor or regular blender will work fine as well.

Bring a saucepan of water up to a boil. Cut the sweet potato into 1-inch dice. Add to the water and cook for 10 minutes or until very tender. Drain well. Measure out 1 packed cup of sweet potato flesh.

While the sweet potato cooks, put the dates in a small bowl or ramekin, cover with boiling water, and let sit for 5 minutes to soften. Drain and set aside.

Combine the sweet potato, dates, cacao powder, salt, vanilla extract, honey, and milk in a blender or food processor. Blend until very smooth.

Divide between 4 ramekins or small serving dishes and chill in the fridge for at least 30 minutes.

Top with whipped cream and berries before serving, if desired.

Serves 4

1 medium sweet potato, peeled

2 Medjool dates, pitted

3 tablespoons raw cacao powder

¼ teaspoon kosher salt

½ teaspoon vanilla extract

1 tablespoon raw honey

6 tablespoons grass-fed whole milk or any plant-based milk

Whipped cream and raspberries (optional)

Strawberry Cheesecake

Strawberry cheesecake over everything! That was my motto growing up. But once I turned my health around, it was *years* before I had cheesecake again. It wasn't until recently that we decided to find a way to create a cheesecake (using as many organic real-food ingredients as possible) that would outmatch the cheesecake experiences I grew up with. This indulgent dessert is the result!

Preheat the oven to 325°F. Lightly grease a 9-inch springform pan with butter.

Mix the graham cracker crumbs and melted butter in a bowl until it is the texture of wet sand and holds together when you squeeze it gently (add another tablespoon of melted butter if it's looking too dry). Transfer to the springform pan and use a flat-bottomed water glass (or similar) to press the base evenly onto the bottom of the pan and 1 to 2 inches up the sides. Transfer to the fridge while you make the filling.

Combine the cream cheese, sugar, and salt in a large bowl or the bowl of a stand mixer. Use a spatula or the paddle attachment to gently mix. Crack in the eggs, mixing after each addition. Mix in the vanilla extract and sour cream.

Transfer the filling to the prepared pan and place the pan on a baking sheet. Bake for 40 minutes; it should still be jiggly in the center when you give it a light shake. Turn off the oven, prop the door open with a folded dish towel to let some of the heat escape, and leave for 15 minutes (see Notes).

Remove to a rack and cool to room temperature. Cover and refrigerate for at least 3 hours, or until completely chilled.

To make the topping, combine the strawberries and sugar in a medium bowl and give them a good mix. Let sit and macerate for 30 minutes before spooning over the entire cheesecake—this can get a little messy but is very beautiful! Or spoon over individual slices.

Serves 8 to 10

CRUST

4 tablespoons unsalted grass-fed butter, melted, plus extra for the pan

1½ cups graham cracker crumbs (from about 7.5 ounces graham crackers, crushed in a food processor—sub gluten-free graham crackers if desired)

FILLING

2 (8-ounce) packages cream cheese, at room temp

¾ cup organic can sugar

¼ teaspoon kosher salt

2 large organic eggs

1 large organic egg yolk

1 teaspoon vanilla extract

½ cup sour cream

TOPPING

2 cups fresh strawberries, cut in halves or quarters

3 tablespoons cane sugar

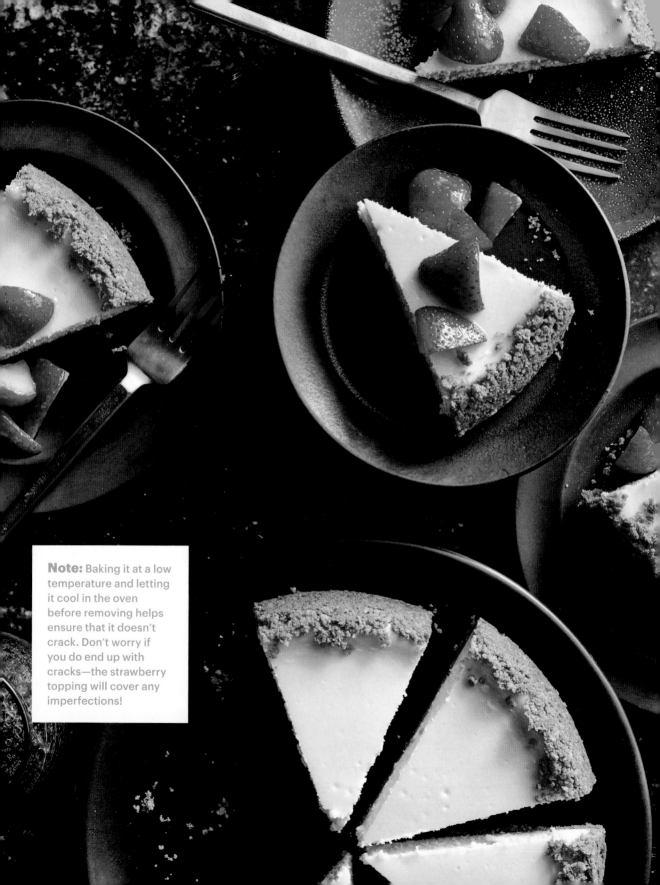

Note: Baking it at a low temperature and letting it cool in the oven before removing helps ensure that it doesn't crack. Don't worry if you do end up with cracks—the strawberry topping will cover any imperfections!

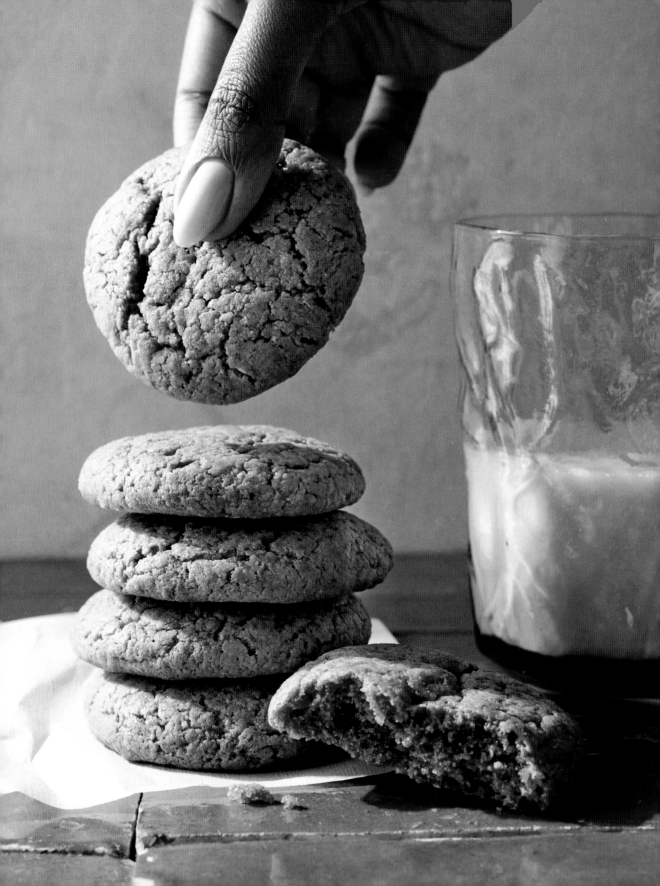

J's Peanut Butter Cookies

I don't know what inspired my son to make peanut butter cookies, but one day, when he was about 16, he went into the kitchen and whipped up some simple, four-ingredient cookies for all of us. This is the culmination of that recipe, staying true to its simplicity.

Preheat the oven to 375°F. Line a baking sheet with parchment paper.

Whisk together the coconut sugar and baking soda. Stir in the peanut butter, mixing to combine. Crack in the egg and mix thoroughly.

Roll into 8 equal balls (about the size of a golf ball) and arrange evenly on the baking sheet. Transfer to the oven and bake for 10 to 12 minutes, turning the pan front to back halfway through, until lightly golden.

Remove from the oven and let cool to room temperature before eating.

Note: The type of peanut butter you use will change the texture a bit—thicker natural peanut butter with no added oils will yield a firmer cookie, for example. But they're great made with any smooth peanut butter.

Makes 8 cookies

⅓ cup coconut sugar

½ teaspoon baking soda

½ cup salted, unsweetened peanut butter (see Note)

1 large organic egg

Dressings
& Sauces

CHAPTER TWELVE Salad dressings and sauces can easily tip the scales in whether a meal is healthy or not. Rather than corrupting our food with low-quality oils typically found in store-bought dressings, we're providing the ultimate health-enriching complements that make your brain and body better with each bite.

Simple and Smart Vinaigrette

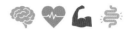

This quick and easy salad dressing features brain- and microbiome-friendly ingredients. Plus, its versatile flavor tastes great with just about any salad veggies you can imagine! One of the highlighted ingredients is apple cider vinegar (ACV). Not only have peer-reviewed studies found ACV helpful in normalizing blood sugar, a randomized trial cited in the journal *Bioscience, Biotechnology & Biochemistry* determined that test subjects including ACV in their diets had improved weight loss, body fat loss, and reduced triglycerides.[15]

Pour the olive oil, vinegar, coconut aminos, lemon juice, and garlic into a bottle, cover tightly, and shake it up. Season to taste with salt and pepper. Shake again before using. The dressing will keep up to 5 days in the refrigerator.

Note: If you'd like to reduce the sharpness of the ACV a bit, a little bit of honey is a welcome addition here!

Makes about 1½ cups

½ cup extra virgin olive oil

½ cup apple cider vinegar (see Note)

¼ cup coconut aminos

¼ cup fresh lemon juice

2 garlic cloves, minced

Sea salt and black pepper

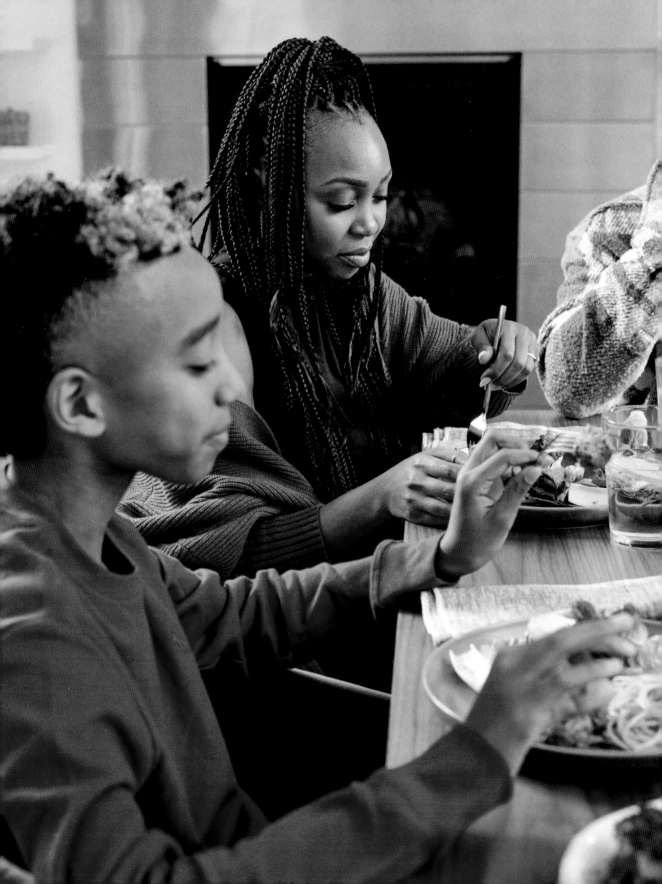

Honey Mustard Dressing

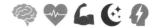

Honey mustard is one of those things that lots of families buy, but it's actually super easy to make yourself! And by making it home, you get to control the quality of the ingredients, which means using the best raw honey you can and ditching any artificial sweeteners or stabilizers often found in commercial versions. I love the balance of spicy and sweet here, but feel free to change up ratios to make it your own!

Whisk the mustard, honey, vinegar, olive oil, garlic powder, and cayenne together in a small bowl. Season with salt and pepper to taste. Use immediately or transfer to a jar and store in the fridge for up to 4 days.

Makes about 1 cup

6 tablespoons Dijon mustard

¼ cup raw honey

2 tablespoons apple cider vinegar

¼ cup olive oil

1 teaspoon garlic powder

Large pinch of cayenne pepper

Sea salt and black pepper

Miso Mayo

Here's a versatile, delicious mayo that supports brain and gut health. I'm definitely a sauce lover, so creating this recipe was a game changer. One of the highlighted ingredients is miso (made from fermented soybeans), which lends a sweet and salty umami flavor. Data published in the journal *Food Science and Technology Research* found that study participants who consumed miso with their meal had improved insulin function and a faster normalization of post-meal blood glucose levels. With a little spicy sriracha and a touch of raw honey, it's an awesome combination you're going to love. You can use it on everything from the Quick and Easy Deviled Eggs (page 250) to Avocado Fries (page 230) to grain bowls and sandwiches. If you like things on the spicier side, just add more sriracha to taste![16]

Whisk together the miso, mayo, honey, and sriracha in a small bowl until fully combined. Use immediately, or transfer to a jar, cover, and store in the fridge for up to a week.

Makes about 1¼ cups

¼ cup white miso

1 cup of your favorite mayo (extra virgin olive oil– or avocado oil–based are ideal!)

2 teaspoons raw honey

2 teaspoons sriracha hot sauce

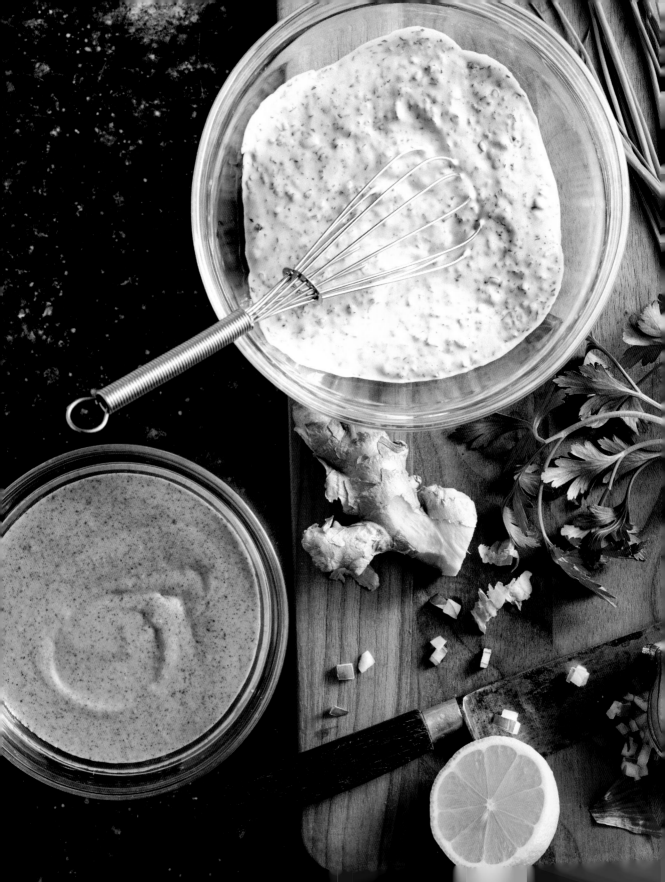

Asante Sana Dressing

I used to think that salad dressing only came in a bottle. Then one day my beautiful mother-in-law made this dressing for me, and I was hooked! Being from Kenya, she taught me that asante sana means "thank you" in Swahili. I'm thankful for this recipe and thankful for her, too.

Put the dates in a small bowl and cover with warm water. Let sit for 5 minutes to soften.

Drain the dates, then combine them with the olive oil, garlic, onion, ginger, almond butter, honey, soy sauce, lemon juice, cayenne, and water in a high-speed blender. Blend on high until smooth, adding more water as needed to reach your desired consistency. (We like it pretty thick but still pourable!)

Use immediately or transfer to a jar, cover, and store in the fridge for up to 4 days.

Note: In addition to salad dressing, this also works as a phenomenal dip! And if you like things spicier, you can add some minced fresh jalapeño, or simply up the amount of cayenne.

Makes about 2 cups

- **2 Medjool dates, pitted**
- **¼ cup extra virgin olive oil**
- **2 garlic cloves, peeled**
- **2 tablespoons minced red onion**
- **1 tablespoon minced fresh ginger**
- **1 cup raw almond butter**
- **1 tablespoon raw honey**
- **1 tablespoon nama shoyu (raw soy sauce) or coconut aminos**
- **Juice of 1 small-medium lemon**
- **¼ teaspoon cayenne pepper**
- **¼ cup water, plus extra as needed**

Superfood Pesto

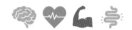

The word pesto originates from a word meaning "to pound," as the traditional method was to pound or crush nuts, spices, salt, cheese, and healthy oils to make this time-honored recipe. Unfortunately, over the years, the quality of conventional pesto has been pounded out of it by using low-quality oils and other subpar ingredients. This version uses phenomenal ingredients, and the taste is delizioso! It's a great spread for wraps (like the Pesto Turkey Wrap on page 180), stirred into pasta or Kelp Noodles (page 236), as a glaze for a protein (like salmon), and mixed with simply roasted vegetables.

Combine the basil, kale and spinach, olive oil, garlic, nuts, and hemp seeds in a blender or food processor. Blend until mostly smooth. Stir in the parm and season to taste with salt and pepper.

Use immediately. Or transfer to a jar or other storage container and top with a thin layer of olive oil to keep the pesto from oxidizing. This will keep in the fridge, covered, for about a week.

Makes about 1 cup

1 cup lightly packed fresh basil leaves, roughly chopped

1 cup lightly packed baby kale and/or spinach, roughly chopped

½ cup olive oil, plus extra for storing

1 large garlic clove, grated or minced

¼ cup raw hazelnuts, walnuts, or almonds, or a mix

2 tablespoons hulled hemp seeds

⅓ cup finely grated parmesan cheese (optional)

Sea salt and black pepper

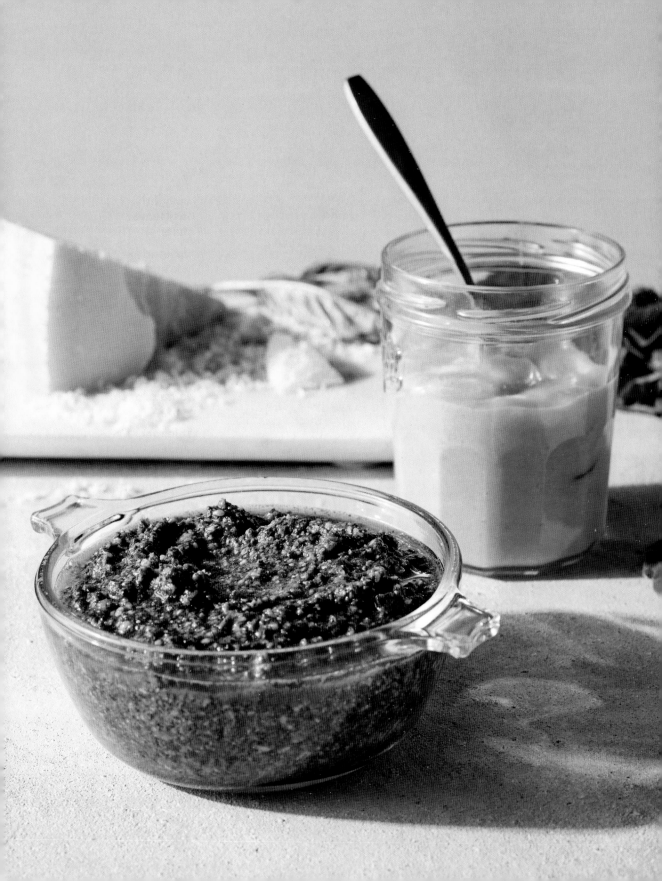

Smarter Ranch Dressing

Conventional ranch dressing simply can't compare to this one! Start with your favorite mayo as the base; I like extra virgin olive oil– or avocado oil–based mayo. Then mix in some time-honored seasonings and fresh herbs to make the very best—and healthiest—ranch dressing you can imagine. So good!

Whisk mayo, onion powder, garlic powder, chives, parsley, and vinegar. Season to taste with salt and pepper. Use immediately, or transfer to a jar, cover, and store in the fridge for up to 4 days.

Makes about 1 cup

1 cup of your favorite mayo

½ teaspoon onion powder

½ teaspoon garlic powder

¼ cup finely chopped fresh chives

¼ cup finely chopped fresh parsley

2 tablespoons red wine vinegar

Sea salt and black pepper

Italian Dressing

This exquisite dressing is a great way to get in some fresh, nutrient-dense herbs and brain-boosting extra virgin olive oil. We love to have it with a big bowl of fresh salad greens, tomato, diced avocado, and radishes (cut into matchsticks), with dulse flakes sprinkled over the top for a truly beautiful salad.

Blend the olive oil, basil, parsley, Italian seasoning, garlic, lemon juice, honey, and salt in a regular or high-speed blender. Pour it into a glass bottle or another container and chill at least 30 minutes before serving. (The longer it sits, the more the flavors get to mingle, and the results are beyond words!) Shake well before pouring it over your salad. Store any leftovers in the fridge for up to 4 days.

Makes about 1½ cups

½ cup extra virgin olive oil

¾ cup lightly packed fresh basil leaves

1 cup lightly packed fresh parsley leaves

3 tablespoons Italian seasoning

1 garlic clove, peeled

Juice of ½ large lemon

¾ teaspoon raw honey

½ teaspoon kosher salt

Acknowledgments

My wife is my best friend, manager of our team, and my greatest inspiration. But she does *not* get excited when she knows I'm working on a new book (she knows very well the work it's going to take!). So, when I saw her get excited about this cookbook I knew this was going to be special.

I want to express my deepest thanks to Anne Stevenson. Thank you for making my life so amazing and thank you for adding your insights (and stunning beauty!) to this book. Immense gratitude to my sons, Jorden Stevenson and Braden Stevenson, for contributing to this project and, of course, eating up all of the recipes.

I'd like to thank the team at Little, Brown Spark for helping to bring this important book to life. Special thank you to Marisa Vigilante for supporting my writing and mission through our third book together. I appreciate you!

Thea Baumann, I can't thank you enough for your recipe genius and helping me to put the puzzle pieces together. Eva Kolenko, what can I say? Your photography skills are out of this world. Thank you for making the experience magical.

Thank you to my agents Scott Hoffman and Steve Troha, *The Model Health Show* Team, and my amazing friends and colleagues who continue to inspire and support me.

Not least of all, I'd like to express my heartfelt gratitude to *The Model Health Show* listeners and all of the wonderful readers of my books. Being a positive force in your life and a part of your incredible story is what continues to push me to be the best that I can possibly be.

Here's to lots of love, excellent health, and amazing food!

Notes

INTRODUCTION

1 *Lancet, The.* "Health Effects of Dietary Risks in 195 Countries." https://www.thelancet.com/journals/lancet/article/PIIS0140-6736(19)30041-8/fulltext

2 *Archives of Pediatrics and Adolescent Medicine.* "Influence of Licensed Spokescharacters and Health Cues on Children's Ratings of Cereal Taste." https://www.ncbi.nlm.nih.gov/pubmed/21383272

3 *PLoS ONE.* "Long-Chain Omega-3 Polyunsaturated Fatty Acid Dietary Intake Is Positively Associated with Bone Mineral Density in Normal and Osteopenic Spanish Women." https://journals.plos.org/plosone/article?id=10.1371/journal.pone.0190539

4 *American Journal of Clinical Nutrition, The.* "Human Plasma and Tissue Alpha-Tocopherol Concentrations in Response to Supplementation with Deuterated Natural and Synthetic Vitamin E." https://pubmed.ncbi.nlm.nih.gov/9537614/

5 *Journal of Cardiology.* "Tropical Fruit Camu-Camu Has Anti-Oxidative and Anti-Inflammatory Properties." https://www.journal-of-cardiology.com/article/S0914-5087(08)00150-0/fulltext

CHAPTER ONE

1 *Archives of Family Medicine.* "Family Dinner and Diet Quality Among Older Children and Adolescents." https://www.ncbi.nlm.nih.gov/pubmed/10728109

2 *Journal of Nutrition Education and Behavior.* "The Association Between Family Meals, TV Viewing During Meals, and Fruit and Vegetables and Soda and Chips Intake Among Latino Children." https://www.ncbi.nlm.nih.gov/pmc/articles/PMC3117953/

3 *BMJ Nutrition and Metabolism.* "Ultra-Processed Foods and Added Sugars in the US Diet: Evidence from a Nationally Representative Cross-Sectional Study." https://bmjopen.bmj.com/content/6/3/e009892

4 *JAMA.* "Trends in Consumption of Ultraprocessed Foods Among US Youths Aged 2–19 Years, 1999–2018." https://jamanetwork.com/journals/jama/fullarticle/2782866

5 *Archives of Family Medicine.* "Too Many Kids Are Too Heavy, Too Young." https://www.hsph.harvard.edu/obesity-prevention-source/obesity-trends/global-obesity-trends-in-children/

6 *National Library of Medicine Global Pediatric Health.* "Childhood and Adolescent Obesity in the United States: A Public Health Concern." https://www.ncbi.nlm.nih.gov/pmc/articles/PMC6887808/

7 *JAMA Network.* "Exploring the Role of Family Functioning in the Association Between Frequency of Family Dinners and Dietary Intake Among Adolescents and Young Adults." https://jamanetwork.com/journals/jamanetworkopen/fullarticle/2715616

8 *Pediatrics.* "Is Frequency of Shared Family Meals Related to the Nutritional Health of Children and Adolescents?" https://www.ncbi.nlm.nih.gov/pmc/articles/PMC3387875/#__ffn_sectitle

9 *Family and Consumer Sciences.* "Work Interference with Dinnertime as a Mediator and Moderator Between Work Hours and Work and Family Outcomes." https://onlinelibrary.wiley.com/doi/abs/10.1177/1077727X08316025

10 *JAMA Internal Medicine.* "When Physicians Counsel About Stress." https://jamanetwork.com/journals/jamainternalmedicine/fullarticle/1392494

11 Harvard Graduate School of Education. "The Benefit of Family Mealtime." https://www.gse.harvard.edu/news/20/04/harvard-edcast-benefit-family-mealtime

12 *PLoS One.* "Genetic Factors Are Not the Major Causes of Chronic Diseases." https://journals.plos.org/plosone/article?id=10.1371/journal.pone.0154387

13 *Science Daily.* "Social Interactions Can Alter Gene Expression in Brain, and Vice Versa." https://www.sciencedaily.com/releases/2008/11/081106153538.htm

14 *Science.* "Genes and Social Behavior." https://www.ncbi.nlm.nih.gov/pmc/articles/PMC3052688/

15 *PLoS Medicine.* "Social Relationships and Mortality Risk: A Meta-analytic Review." https://journals.plos.org/plosmedicine/article/authors?id=10.1371/journal.pmed.1000316

16 Centers for Disease Control. "Loneliness and Social Isolation Linked to Serious Health Conditions." https://www.cdc.gov/aging/publications/features/lonely-older-adults.html

17 American Psychiatric Association. "New Survey Shows Increasing Loneliness, Including on the Job." https://www.psychiatry.org/News-room/APA-Blogs/New-Survey-Shows-Increasing-Loneliness-on-the-Job

18 *University of Chicago Press Journals, The.* "Brain Drain: The Mere Presence of One's Own Smartphone Reduces Available Cognitive Capacity." https://www.journals.uchicago.edu/doi/full/10.1086/691462

19 American Psychological Association. "The Mere Presence of a Cell Phone May Be Distracting: Implications for Attention and Task Performance." https://psycnet.apa.org/doiLanding?doi=10.1027%2F1864-9335%2Fa000216

20 *BMC Nutrition Journal.* "Association Between Eating Behaviour and Diet Quality: Eating Alone Vs. Eating with Others." https://nutritionj.biomedcentral.com/articles/10.1186/s12937-018-0424-0

CHAPTER TWO

1 *American Journal of Clinical Nutrition, The.* "Is the Degree of Food Processing and Convenience Linked with the Nutritional Quality of Foods Purchased by US Households." https://academic.oup.com/ajcn/article/101/6/1251/4626878

2 *Forbes.* "America's Largest Private Companies: Cargill Is Back at No. 1." https://www.forbes.com/sites/andreamurphy/2021/11/23/americas-largest-private-companies-cargill-is-back-at-no-1/?sh=5076a1932b70; Cargill. "Sugar When You Need It." https://www.cargill.com/food-beverage/na/sugar

3 *Advances in Nutrition.* "Adaptation of the Gut Microbiota to Modern Dietary Sugars and Sweeteners." https://academic.oup.com/advances/article/11/3/616/5614218

4 *Metabolic Syndrome and Related Disorders.* "Prevalence of Optimal Metabolic Health in American Adults: National Health and Nutrition Examination Survey 2009–2016." https://www.liebertpub.com/doi/10.1089/met.2018.0105

5 *Interdisciplinary Toxicology.* "Glyphosate, Pathways to Modern Diseases II: Celiac Sprue and Gluten Intolerance." https://www.ncbi.nlm.nih.gov/pmc/articles/PMC3945755/

6 WHO International Agency for Research on Cancer. "IARC Monographs Volume 112: Evaluation of Five Organophosphate Insecticides and Herbicides." https://www.iarc.who.int/wp-content/uploads/2018/07/MonographVolume112-1.pdf

7 *Journal of Nutritional Biochemistry, The.* "High-Fructose Diet Leads to Visceral Adiposity and Hypothalamic Leptin Resistance in Male Rats—Do Glucocorticoids Play a Role?" https://www.sciencedirect.com/science/article/abs/pii/S0955286314000023?via%3Dihub

8 *American Journal of Clinical Nutrition, The.* "Consumption of High-Fructose Corn Syrup in Beverages May Play a Role in the Epidemic of Obesity." https://academic.oup.com/ajcn/article/79/4/537/4690128

9 *Journal of Nutrition, The.* "Greater Fructose Consumption Is Associated with Cardiometabolic Risk Markers and Visceral Adiposity in Adolescents." https://www.ncbi.nlm.nih.gov/pmc/articles/PMC3260058/

10 *Stroke.* "Sugar- and Artificially-Sweetened Beverages and the Risks of Incident Stroke and Dementia: A Prospective Cohort Study." https://www.ncbi.nlm.nih.gov/pmc/articles/PMC5405737/

11 American Diabetes Society. "Sucralose Affects Glycemic and Hormonal Responses to an Oral Glucose Load." https://diabetesjournals.org/care/article/36/9/2530/37872/Sucralose-Affects-Glycemic-and-Hormonal-Responses

12 *Advances in Nutrition.* "Adaptation of the Gut Microbiota to Modern Dietary Sugars and Sweeteners." https://academic.oup.com/advances/article/11/3/616/5614218

13 *Frontiers in Physiology.* "Gut Microbiome Response to Sucralose and Its Potential Role in Inducing Liver Inflammation in Mice." https://www.ncbi.nlm.nih.gov/pmc/articles/PMC5522834/

14 *Nutrients.* "Potential Effects of Sucralose and Saccharin on Gut Microbiota: A Review." https://www.mdpi.com/2072-6643/14/8/1682

15 *BMC Biochemistry.* "Digested Wheat Gluten Inhibits Binding Between Leptin and Its Receptor." https://bmcbiochem.biomedcentral.com/articles/10.1186/s12858-015-0032-y

16 *Nutrients.* "The Dietary Intake of Wheat and Other Cereal Grains and Their Role in Inflammation." https://www.ncbi.nlm.nih.gov/pmc/articles/PMC3705319/

17 Environmental Working Group. "Glyphosate Contamination in Food Goes Far Beyond Oat Products." https://www.ewg.org/news-insights/news/glyphosate-contamination-food-goes-far-beyond-oat-products

18 Environmental Working Group. "Roundup for Breakfast, Part 2: In New Tests, Weed Killer Found in All Kids' Cereals Sampled." https://www.ewg.org/news-insights/news-release/2018/10/roundup-breakfast-part-2-new-tests-weed-killer-found-all-kids

19 *JAMA Internal Medicine.* "Association of Frequency of Organic Food Consumption with Cancer Risk Findings from the NutriNet-Santé Prospective Cohort Study." https://jamanetwork.com/journals/jamainternalmedicine/fullarticle/2707948

20 Shanahan, Catherine. *The Fat Burn Fix.* https://us.macmillan.com/books/9781250114495/thefatburnfix

21 Shanahan, Catherine. "Seed Oils: Q & A for Your Health." https://drcate.com/seed-oils-questions-answers-for-your-health/

22 *BMJ: Open Heart.* "Omega-6 Vegetable Oils as a Driver of Coronary Heart Disease: The Oxidized Linoleic Acid Hypothesis." https://openheart.bmj.com/content/5/2/e000898

23 *Inhalation Toxicology.* "Increased Levels of Oxidative DNA Damage Attributable to Cooking-Oil Fumes Exposure Among Cooks." https://pubmed.ncbi.nlm.nih.gov/19225966/

24 *Environmental Science and Pollution Research International.* "Characteristics of PAHs from Deep-Frying and Frying Cooking Fumes." https://pubmed.ncbi.nlm.nih.gov/26066859/

25 University of California, Riverside. "America's Most Widely Consumed Cooking Oil Causes Genetic Changes in the Brain." https://www.universityofcalifornia.edu/news/americas-most-widely-consumed-cooking-oil-causes-genetic-changes-brain

26 *Endocrinology.* "Dysregulation of Hypothalamic Gene Expression and the Oxytocinergic System by Soybean Oil Diets in Male Mice." https://academic.oup.com/endo/article/161/2/bqz044/5698148?login=false

27 *Journal of the National Cancer Institute.* "Serum Concentrations of Per- and Polyfluoroalkyl Substances and Risk of Renal Cell Carcinoma." https://pubmed.ncbi.nlm.nih.gov/32944748/

28 *Environmental Science and Pollution Research International.* "PTFE-Coated Non-Stick Cookware and Toxicity Concerns: A Perspective." https://pubmed.ncbi.nlm.nih.gov/28913736/

29 *Nutrition Journal.* "Trends in US Home Food Preparation and Consumption: Analysis of National Nutrition Surveys and Time Use Studies from 1965–1966 to 2007–2008." https://pubmed.ncbi.nlm.nih.gov/23577692/

30 *Tufts University Health & Nutrition Letter.* "28% of Americans Can't Cook." https://www.nutritionletter.tufts.edu/general-nutrition/28-of-americans-cant-cook/

31 *Frontiers in Bioscience.* "Xenoestrogen Exposure and Mechanisms of Endocrine Disruption." https://www.ncbi.nlm.nih.gov/pubmed/12456297

32 *Environmental Research.* "Large Effects from Small Exposures. II. The Importance of Positive Controls in Low-Dose Research on Bisphenol A." https://www.sciencedirect.com/science/article/abs/pii/S0013935105001258?via%3Dihub

33 *Fertility and Sterility.* "Urine Bisphenol-A (BPA) Level in Relation to Semen Quality." https://www.ncbi.nlm.nih.gov/pubmed/21035116

34 *Journal of Clinical Endocrinology and Metabolism, The.* "Urinary Bisphenol A (BPA) Concentration Associates with Obesity and Insulin Resistance." https://www.ncbi.nlm.nih.gov/pubmed/22090277

35 *Environmental Health Perspectives.* "Bisphenol S and F: A Systematic Review and Comparison of the Hormonal Activity of Bisphenol A Substitutes." https://www.ncbi.nlm.nih.gov/m/pubmed/25775505/

36 *International Journal of Obesity.* "The Influence of 15-Week Exercise Training on Dietary Patterns Among Young Adults." https://www.nature.com/articles/s41366-018-0299-3

37 *Journal of Science & Medicine in Sport.* "Effects of Physical Activity on Executive Functions, Attention and Academic Performance in Preadolescent Children." https://pubmed.ncbi.nlm.nih.gov/29054748/

38 *Oxidative Medicine and Cellular Longevity.* "Exercise Modifies the Gut Microbiota with Positive Health Effects." https://www.ncbi.nlm.nih.gov/pmc/articles/PMC5357536/

39 *Journal of Physiology and Pharmacology.* "Stress and the Gut: Pathophysiology, Clinical Consequences, Diagnostic Approach and Treatment Options." https://pubmed.ncbi.nlm.nih.gov/22314561/

40 *Gastroenterology.* "Burden of Gastrointestinal Disease in the United States: 2012 Update." https://www.ncbi.nlm.nih.gov/pmc/articles/PMC3480553/

41 *Journal of Physiology, The.* "Role of the Vagus Nerve in the Development and Treatment of Diet-Induced Obesity." https://physoc.onlinelibrary.wiley.com/doi/full/10.1113/JP271538

42 *Annals of the New York Academy of Sciences.* "Hypothalamic Inflammation: A Double-Edged Sword to Nutritional Diseases." https://www.ncbi.nlm.nih.gov/pmc/articles/PMC4389774/

43 *Visceral Medicine.* "The Pathophysiology of Malabsorption." https://www.karger.com/Article/FullText/364794

44 *BioMed Research International.* "Mastication as a Stress-Coping Behavior." https://pubmed.ncbi.nlm.nih.gov/26090453/

CHAPTER THREE

1 *Biology of Sport.* "Effects of Supplementation with Acai Berry-Based Juice Blend on the Blood Antioxidant Defense Capacity and Lipid Profile in Junior Hurdlers. A Pilot Study." https://www.ncbi.nlm.nih.gov/pmc/articles/PMC4447763/

2 *Nutritional Neuroscience.* "Dietary Supplementation with the Polyphenol-Rich Açaí Pulps Improves Cognition in Aged Rats and Attenuates Inflammatory Signaling in BV-2 Microglial Cells." https://pubmed.ncbi.nlm.nih.gov/26618555/

3 *University of Michigan–Science Daily.* "Blueberries May Help Reduce Belly Fat, Diabetes Risk." https://www.sciencedaily.com/releases/2009/04/090419170112.htm

4 *Harvard Health Publishing.* "Eat Blueberries and Strawberries Three Times Per Week." https://www.health.harvard.edu/heart-health/eat-blueberries-and-strawberries-three-times-per-week

5 *Journal of Nutrition, The.* "Bioactives in Blueberries Improve Insulin Sensitivity in Obese, Insulin-Resistant Men and Women." https://www.ncbi.nlm.nih.gov/pmc/articles/PMC3139238/#__ffn_sectitle

6 *Journal of Agricultural and Food Chemistry.* "Six-Week Consumption of a Wild Blueberry Powder Drink Increases Bifidobacteria in the Human Gut." https://www.ncbi.nlm.nih.gov/pubmed/22060186

7 *International Journal of Food Sciences and Nutrition.* "Inhibitory Effects of Sweet Cherry Anthocyanins on the Obesity Development in C57BL/6 Mice." https://www.ncbi.nlm.nih.gov/pubmed/24224922

8 *European Journal of Nutrition.* "Effect of Tart Cherry Juice on Melatonin Levels and Enhanced Sleep Quality." https://pubmed.ncbi.nlm.nih.gov/22038497/

9 *Medicinal Chemistry.* "Practical Application of Antidiabetic Efficacy of Lycium Barbarum Polysaccharide in Patients with Type 2 Diabetes." https://www.ncbi.nlm.nih.gov/pmc/articles/PMC4475782/#!po=1.11111

10 *Neural Regeneration Research.* "Efficacy of Lycium Barbarum Polysaccharide in Adolescents with Subthreshold Depression: Interim Analysis of a Randomized Controlled Study." https://pubmed.ncbi.nlm.nih.gov/34916444/

11 *Current Developments in Nutrition.* "Effects of Avocado Consumption on Abdominal Adiposity and Glucose Tolerance." https://www.ncbi.nlm.nih.gov/pmc/articles/PMC6578444/

12 *Journal of Nutrition, The.* "Avocado Consumption Alters Gastrointestinal Bacteria Abundance and Microbial Metabolite Concentrations Among Adults with Overweight or Obesity: A Randomized Controlled Trial." https://www.ncbi.nlm.nih.gov/pmc/articles/PMC8030699/

13 *Frontiers in Endocrinology.* "Recurrent Hypoglycemia Increases Anxiety and Amygdala Norepinephrine Release During Subsequent Hypoglycemia." https://www.ncbi.nlm.nih.gov/pmc/articles/PMC4653740/

14 *Nutrients.* "Using the Avocado to Test the Satiety Effects of a Fat-Fiber Combination in Place of Carbohydrate Energy in a Breakfast Meal in Overweight and Obese Men and Women: A Randomized Clinical Trial." https://www.ncbi.nlm.nih.gov/pmc/articles/PMC6567160/

15 *Molecular Nutrition & Food Research.* "Avocatin B Protects Against Lipotoxicity and Improves Insulin Sensitivity in Diet-Induced Obesity." https://onlinelibrary.wiley.com/doi/10.1002/mnfr.201900688

16 *Immunity & Aging.* "Nutraceutical Effects of Table Green Olives: A Pilot Study with Nocellara Del Belice Olives." https://pubmed.ncbi.nlm.nih.gov/27053940/

17 *Nutrition Reviews.* "Effect of Diet on Adiponectin Levels in Blood." https://www.ncbi.nlm.nih.gov/pubmed/21967160/

18 *BioImpacts.* "Protective Mechanisms of *Cucumis sativus* in Diabetes-Related Models of Oxidative Stress and Carbonyl Stress." https://pubmed.ncbi.nlm.nih.gov/27340622/

19 *Gut.* "Effects of Targeted Delivery of Propionate to the Human Colon on Appetite Regulation, Body Weight Maintenance and Adiposity in Overweight Adults." https://www.ncbi.nlm.nih.gov/pubmed/25500202

20 *International Journal of Molecular Sciences.* "Isothiocyanates Are Promising Compounds Against Oxidative Stress, Neuroinflammation and Cell Death That May Benefit Neurodegeneration in Parkinson's Disease." https://www.ncbi.nlm.nih.gov/pmc/articles/PMC5037733/

21 *Anticancer Agents in Medicinal Chemistry.* "Natural Products as Aromatase Inhibitors." https://www.ncbi.nlm.nih.gov/pmc/articles/PMC3074486/

22 *Primary Care Diabetes.* "Consumption of Citrus and Cruciferous Vegetables with Incident Type 2 Diabetes Mellitus Based on a Meta-Analysis of Prospective Study." https://pubmed.ncbi.nlm.nih.gov/26778708/

23 *Appetite*. "Dietary Nutrients Associated with Short and Long Sleep Duration. Data from a Nationally Representative Sample." https://www.ncbi.nlm.nih.gov/pmc/articles/PMC3703747/

24 *PLoS One*. "Serum Nutritional Biomarkers and Their Associations with Sleep Among US Adults in Recent National Surveys." https://journals.plos.org/plosone/article?id=10.1371/journal.pone.0103490

25 *Nutrition Research*. "Fermented Kimchi Reduces Body Weight and Improves Metabolic Parameters in Overweight and Obese Patients." https://www.ncbi.nlm.nih.gov/pubmed/21745625

26 *Appetite*. "Body Weight Loss, Reduced Urge for Palatable Food and Increased Release of GLP-1 Through Daily Supplementation with Green-Plant Membranes for Three Months in Overweight Women." https://www.ncbi.nlm.nih.gov/pubmed/24993695

27 *Neurology*. "Nutrients and Bioactives in Green Leafy Vegetables and Cognitive Decline." https://n.neurology.org/content/90/3/e214

28 *Food Science and Human Wellness*. "Dietary Seaweeds and Obesity." https://www.sciencedirect.com/science/article/pii/S2213453015000439

29 *International Journal of Obesity*. "An Intervention Study of the Effects of Calcium Intake on Fecal Fat Excretion, Energy Metabolism and Adipose Tissue MRNA Expression of Lipid-Metabolism Related Proteins." https://www.ncbi.nlm.nih.gov/pubmed/17579637

30 *Journal of Agricultural and Food Chemistry*. "The Modulatory Effect of Anthocyanins from Purple Sweet Potato on Human Intestinal Microbiota In Vitro." https://pubmed.ncbi.nlm.nih.gov/26975278/

31 *Wake Forest University–Science Daily*. "Soluble Fiber Strikes a Blow to Belly Fat." https://onlinelibrary.wiley.com/doi/full/10.1038/oby.2011.171

32 *Nutrients*. "White Sweet Potato as Meal Replacement for Overweight White-Collar Workers: A Randomized Controlled Trial." https://www.mdpi.com/2072-6643/11/1/165/htm

33 *Archives of Pharmacal Research*. "Antioxidant and Memory Enhancing Effects of Purple Sweet Potato Anthocyanin and Cordyceps Mushroom Extract." https://pubmed.ncbi.nlm.nih.gov/14609130/

34 *International Journal of Obesity*. "Egg Breakfast Enhances Weight Loss." https://www.ncbi.nlm.nih.gov/pubmed/18679412

35 *Nutrients*. "Consuming Two Eggs per Day, as Compared to an Oatmeal Breakfast, Decreases Plasma Ghrelin While Maintaining the LDL/HDL Ratio." https://www.ncbi.nlm.nih.gov/pmc/articles/PMC5331520/

36 *Journal of the American College of Nutrition*. "Nutritional Importance of Choline for Brain Development." https://www.ncbi.nlm.nih.gov/pubmed/15640516/

37 *Nutrients*. "Consuming Two Eggs per Day, as Compared to an Oatmeal Breakfast, Decreases Plasma Ghrelin while Maintaining the LDL/HDL Ratio." https://www.ncbi.nlm.nih.gov/pmc/articles/PMC5331520/

38 *Food & Nutrition Research*. "Role of Poultry Meat in a Balanced Diet Aimed at Maintaining Health and Wellbeing: An Italian Consensus Document." https://www.ncbi.nlm.nih.gov/pmc/articles/PMC4462824/

39 *Obesity Science & Practice*. "Equivalent Reductions in Body Weight During the Beef WISE Study: Beef's Role in Weight Improvement, Satisfaction and Energy." https://pubmed.ncbi.nlm.nih.gov/29071106/

40 *European Journal of Clinical Nutrition*. "Effect of Zinc Supplementation on Mood States in Young Women." https://www.nature.com/articles/ejcn2009158

41 *Neuropsychopharmacology*. "The Sleep-Promoting and Hypothermic Effects of Glycine Are Mediated by NMDA Receptors in the Suprachiasmatic Nucleus." https://www.ncbi.nlm.nih.gov/pmc/articles/PMC4397399/

42 *British Journal of Nutrition, The*. "Consumption of Dairy Foods in Relation to Impaired Glucose Metabolism and Type 2 Diabetes Mellitus: The Maastricht Study." https://pubmed.ncbi.nlm.nih.gov/26907098/

43 *American Journal of Clinical Nutrition, The*. "Dairy Consumption in Association with Weight Change and Risk of Becoming Overweight or Obese in Middle-Aged and Older Women." https://pubmed.ncbi.nlm.nih.gov/26912496/

44 *University of Maryland School of Medicine–Science Daily*. "Probiotic-Containing Yogurt Protects Against Microbiome Changes That Lead to Antibiotic-Induced Diarrhea." https://www.sciencedaily.com/releases/2021/09/210914184820.htm

45 *Journal of Nutrition, The*. "A Comparison of the Effects of Beef, Chicken and Fish Protein on Satiety and Amino Acid Profiles in Lean Male Subjects." https://www.ncbi.nlm.nih.gov/pubmed/1542005

46 *International Journal of Obesity*. "Randomized Trial of Weight-Loss-Diets for Young Adults Varying in Fish and Fish Oil Content." https://www.ncbi.nlm.nih.gov/pubmed/17502874

47 *American Journal of Psychiatry, The*. "Vitamin B(12) Deficiency and Depression in Physically Disabled Older Women: Epidemiologic Evidence from the Women's Health and Aging Study." https://pubmed.ncbi.nlm.nih.gov/10784463/

48 *Evidence-Based Complementary and Alternative Medicine*. "Spirulina in Clinical Practice: Evidence-Based Human Applications." https://www.hindawi.com/journals/ecam/2011/531053/

49 *PLoS One*. "Spirulina Promotes Stem Cell Genesis and Protects against LPS Induced Declines in Neural Stem Cell Proliferation." https://www.ncbi.nlm.nih.gov/pmc/articles/PMC2864748/

50 *European Review for Medical and Pharmacological Sciences*. "Effects of Spirulina Consumption on Body Weight, Blood Pressure, and Endothelial Function in Overweight Hypertensive Caucasians: A Double-Blind, Placebo-Controlled, Randomized Trial." https://www.ncbi.nlm.nih.gov/pubmed/26813468

51 *Journal of Nutrition, The*. "Whey Protein But Not Soy Protein Supplementation Alters Body Weight and Composition in Free-Living Overweight and Obese Adults." https://pubmed.ncbi.nlm.nih.gov/21677076/

52 *American Journal of Clinical Nutrition, The*. "Whey Protein Rich in Alpha-Lactalbumin Increases the Ratio of Plasma Tryptophan to the Sum of the Other Large Neutral Amino Acids and Improves Cognitive Performance in Stress-Vulnerable Subjects." https://pubmed.ncbi.nlm.nih.gov/12036812/

53 *Nutrition*. "Moderate Consumption of Fatty Fish Reduces Diastolic Blood Pressure in Overweight and Obese European Young Adults During Energy Restriction." https://pubmed.ncbi.nlm.nih.gov/19487105/

54 *Rush University Medical Center–Science Daily.* "Stave Off Cognitive Decline with Seafood." https://www.sciencedaily.com/releases/2016/05/160510124831.htm

55 *Translational Psychiatry.* "Meta-Analysis and Meta-Regression of Omega-3 Polyunsaturated Fatty Acid Supplementation for Major Depressive Disorder." https://www.ncbi.nlm.nih.gov/pmc/articles/PMC4872453/

56 *Journal of Research in Medical Sciences.* "The Effect of Almonds on Anthropometric Measurements and Lipid Profile in Overweight and Obese Females in a Weight Reduction Program: A Randomized Controlled Clinical Trial." https://www.ncbi.nlm.nih.gov/pmc/articles/PMC4116579/

57 *Journal of Nutrition, The.* "Almonds Decrease Postprandial Glycemia, Insulinemia, and Oxidative Damage in Healthy Individuals." https://pubmed.ncbi.nlm.nih.gov/17116708/

58 *Nutrition, Metabolism, and Cardiovascular Diseases.* "Salba-chia in the Treatment of Overweight and Obese Patients with Type 2 Diabetes: A Double-Blind Randomized Controlled Trial." https://pubmed.ncbi.nlm.nih.gov/28089080/

59 *Nutrients.* "Soluble Extracts from Chia Seed Affect Brush Border Membrane Functionality, Morphology and Intestinal Bacterial Populations In Vivo." https://www.ncbi.nlm.nih.gov/pmc/articles/PMC6835468/

60 *American Journal of Clinical Nutrition, The.* "Prebiotic Evaluation of Cocoa-Derived Flavanols in Healthy Humans by Using a Randomized, Controlled, Double-Blind, Crossover Intervention Study." https://pubmed.ncbi.nlm.nih.gov/21068351/

61 *Columbia University Medical Center–Science Daily.* "Dietary Cocoa Flavanols Reverse Age-Related Memory Decline in Healthy Older Adults." https://www.sciencedaily.com/releases/2014/10/141026195046.htm

62 *International Journal of Health Sciences.* "Effects of Chocolate Intake on Perceived Stress: A Controlled Clinical Study." https://pubmed.ncbi.nlm.nih.gov/25780358/

63 *Inflammation.* "Gamma-Linolenic Acid Inhibits Inflammatory Responses by Regulating NF-Kappab and AP-1 Activation in Lipopolysaccharide-Induced RAW 264.7 Macrophages." https://pubmed.ncbi.nlm.nih.gov/19842026/

64 *American Journal of Physiology.* "Effect of Dietary Hempseed Intake on Cardiac Ischemia-Reperfusion Injury." https://journals.physiology.org/doi/full/10.1152/ajpregu.00661.2006

65 *Nutrients.* "Influence of Tryptophan and Serotonin on Mood and Cognition with a Possible Role of the Gut-Brain Axis." https://www.ncbi.nlm.nih.gov/pmc/articles/PMC4728667/

66 *Journal of Diabetes and Its Complications.* "Antidiabetic Effect of Flax and Pumpkin Seed Mixture Powder: Effect on Hyperlipidemia and Antioxidant Status in Alloxan Diabetic Rats." https://www.ncbi.nlm.nih.gov/pubmed/21106396

67 *European Journal of Nutrition.* "In Vitro Starch Digestibility and In Vivo Glucose Response of Gluten-Free Foods and Their Gluten Counterparts." https://pubmed.ncbi.nlm.nih.gov/15309439/

68 *Plant Foods for Human Nutrition.* "Effect of Quinoa Seeds in Diet on Some Biochemical Parameters and Essential Elements in Blood of High Fructose-Fed Rats." https://link.springer.com/article/10.1007/s11130-010-0197-x

69 *Neurochemical Research.* "Protective Effects of Walnut Extract Against Amyloid Beta Peptide-Induced Cell Death and Oxidative Stress in PC12 Cells." https://www.ncbi.nlm.nih.gov/pmc/articles/PMC3183245/

70 *Journal of Nutrition, Health, and Aging, The.* "A Cross Sectional Study of the Association Between Walnut Consumption and Cognitive Function Among Adult US Populations Represented in NHANES." https://link.springer.com/article/10.1007/s12603-014-0569-2

71 *American Journal of Clinical Nutrition, The.* "α-Linolenic Acid and Risk of Cardiovascular Disease: A Systematic Review and Meta-Analysis." https://pubmed.ncbi.nlm.nih.gov/23076616/

72 *Nutrients.* "A Walnut-Enriched Diet Affects Gut Microbiome in Healthy Caucasian Subjects: A Randomized, Controlled Trial." https://pubmed.ncbi.nlm.nih.gov/29470389/

73 *Experimental and Therapeutic Medicine.* "Antistress and Antioxidant Effects of Virgin Coconut Oil In Vivo." https://www.ncbi.nlm.nih.gov/pmc/articles/PMC4247320/

74 *PLoS One.* "Is Butter Back? A Systematic Review and Meta-Analysis of Butter Consumption and Risk of Cardiovascular Disease, Diabetes, and Total Mortality." https://www.ncbi.nlm.nih.gov/pmc/articles/PMC4927102

75 *Journal of the Pakistan Medical Association, The.* "Anti-Inflammatory Effects of Conjugated Linoleic Acid on Young Athletic Males." https://www.ncbi.nlm.nih.gov/pubmed/26968277

76 *Journal of Dairy Science.* "Conjugated Linoleic Acid Content of Milk from Cows Fed Different Diets." https://www.journalofdairyscience.org/article/S0022-0302(99)75458-5/pdf

77 *International Journal of Obesity and Related Metabolic Disorders.* "Value of VLCD Supplementation with Medium Chain Triglycerides." https://www.ncbi.nlm.nih.gov/pubmed/11571605

78 *Diabetes.* "Medium-Chain Fatty Acids Improve Cognitive Function in Intensively Treated Type 1 Diabetic Patients and Support In Vitro Synaptic Transmission During Acute Hypoglycemia." https://www.ncbi.nlm.nih.gov/pmc/articles/PMC2671041/#__ffn_sectitle

79 *Annals of the New York Academy of Sciences.* "Can Ketones Compensate for Deteriorating Brain Glucose Uptake During Aging? Implications for the Risk and Treatment of Alzheimer's Disease." https://www.ncbi.nlm.nih.gov/pubmed/26766547

80 *ACS Chemical Neuroscience.* "Oleocanthal Enhances Amyloid-β Clearance from the Brains of TgSwDI Mice and In Vitro Across a Human Blood-Brain Barrier Model." https://www.ncbi.nlm.nih.gov/pmc/articles/PMC4653763/

81 *American Journal of Clinical Nutrition, The.* "The 2-Monoacylglycerol Moiety of Dietary Fat Appears to Be Responsible for the Fat-Induced Release of GLP-1 in Humans." https://www.ncbi.nlm.nih.gov/pubmed/26178726

82 *European Journal of Nutrition.* "Consumption of Extra Virgin Olive Oil Improves Body Composition and Blood Pressure in Women with Excess Body Fat: A Randomized, Double-Blinded, Placebo-Controlled Clinical Trial." https://www.ncbi.nlm.nih.gov/pubmed/28808791

83 *International Journal of Environmental Research and Public Health.* "Effects of Dehydration and Rehydration on Cognitive Performance and Mood Among Male College Students in Cangzhou, China: A Self-Controlled Trial." https://www.ncbi.nlm.nih.gov/pubmed/31146326

84 *Journal of Clinical Endocrinology and Metabolism, The.* "Water-Induced Thermogenesis." https://academic.oup.com/jcem/article/88/12/6015/2661518?login=false

85 *Practical Neurology.* "Effects of Coffee/Caffeine on Brain Health and Disease: What Should I Tell My Patients?" https://www.ncbi.nlm.nih.gov/pubmed/26677204

86 *Stanford Medicine.* "Caffeine May Counter Age-Related Inflammation." https://med.stanford.edu/news/all-news/2017/01/caffeine-may-counter-age-related-inflammation-study-finds.html

87 *Nutrition.* "Habitual Coffee Consumption Inversely Associated with Metabolic Syndrome-Related Biomarkers Involving Adiponectin." https://www.ncbi.nlm.nih.gov/pubmed/23602227

88 *Scientific Reports.* "Caffeine Exposure Induces Browning Features in Adipose Tissue In Vitro and In Vivo." https://www.nature.com/articles/s41598-019-45540-1

89 *Journal of Health Science.* "Effects of Combination of Regular Exercise and Tea Catechins Intake on Energy Expenditure in Humans." http://jhs.pharm.or.jp/data/51(2)/51_233.pdf

90 *Physiology & Behavior.* "Effectiveness of Green Tea on Weight Reduction in Obese Thais: A Randomized, Controlled Trial." https://www.ncbi.nlm.nih.gov/pubmed/18006026

91 *Journal of Functional Foods.* "Theaflavin, a Black Tea Polyphenol, Stimulates Lipolysis Associated with the Induction of Mitochondrial Uncoupling Proteins and AMPK–Foxo3a–MnSOD Pathway in 3T3-L1 Adipocytes." https://www.sciencedirect.com/science/article/abs/pii/S1756464615002716

92 *Cochrane Database of Systematic Reviews.* "Green and Black Tea for the Primary Prevention of Cardiovascular Disease." https://www.cochranelibrary.com/cdsr/doi/10.1002/14651858.CD009934.pub2/full

93 *Phytomedicine.* "Effects of Fermented Rooibos (*Aspalathus linearis*) on Adipocyte Differentiation." https://www.ncbi.nlm.nih.gov/pubmed/24060217

94 *Brain Topography.* "The Effects of L-Theanine on Alpha-Band Oscillatory Brain Activity During a Visuo-Spatial Attention Task." https://www.ncbi.nlm.nih.gov/pubmed/18841456

95 *Journal of Alzheimer's Disease.* "Interaction of Cinnamaldehyde and Epicatechin with Tau: Implications of Beneficial Effects in Modulating Alzheimer's Disease Pathogenesis." https://www.ncbi.nlm.nih.gov/pubmed/23531502

96 *Journal of Neuroimmune Pharmacology.* "Cinnamon Converts Poor Learning Mice to Good Learners: Implications for Memory Improvement." https://link.springer.com/article/10.1007%2Fs11481-016-9693-6

97 *Diabetes, Obesity & Metabolism.* "The Potential of Cinnamon to Reduce Blood Glucose Levels in Patients with Type 2 Diabetes and Insulin Resistance." https://pubmed.ncbi.nlm.nih.gov/19930003/

98 *Ohio State University, The.* "Lashing Out at Your Spouse? Check Your Blood Sugar." https://news.osu.edu/lashing-out-at-your-spouse-check-your-blood-sugar/

99 *Antioxidants.* "Potential Health Benefit of Garlic Based on Human Intervention Studies." https://www.mdpi.com/2076-3921/9/7/619

100 *Food Science and Human Wellness.* "Study on Prebiotic Effectiveness of Neutral Garlic Fructan In Vitro." https://www.sciencedirect.com/science/article/pii/S2213453013000311

101 *Drug and Chemical Toxicology.* "Beneficial Effects of Garlic on Learning and Memory Deficits and Brain Tissue Damages Induced by Lead Exposure During Juvenile Rat Growth Is Comparable to the Effect of Ascorbic Acid." https://www.ncbi.nlm.nih.gov/pubmed/27387089

102 *Carbohydrate Polymers.* "Structural Analyses and Immunomodulatory Properties of Fructo-Oligosaccharides from Onion." https://pubmed.ncbi.nlm.nih.gov/25498616/

103 *Gut.* "Effects of Targeted Delivery of Propionate to the Human Colon on Appetite Regulation, Body Weight Maintenance and Adiposity in Overweight Adults." https://www.ncbi.nlm.nih.gov/pubmed/25500202

104 *British Journal of Nutrition, The.* "Effects of a Quercetin-Rich Onion Skin Extract on 24 H Ambulatory Blood Pressure and Endothelial Function in Overweight-To-Obese Patients with (Pre-) Hypertension." https://pubmed.ncbi.nlm.nih.gov/26328470/

105 *Nutrients.* "A Review on the Protective Effects of Honey Against Metabolic Syndrome." https://www.ncbi.nlm.nih.gov/pmc/articles/PMC6115915/

106 *Evidence-Based Complementary and Alternative Medicine.* "Neurological Effects of Honey: Current and Future Prospects." https://www.ncbi.nlm.nih.gov/pmc/articles/PMC4020454/

107 *Pediatrics.* "Effect of Honey on Nocturnal Cough and Sleep Quality: A Double-Blind, Randomized, Placebo-Controlled Study." https://www.ncbi.nlm.nih.gov/pubmed/22869830

108 *Metabolism.* "Low-Salt Diet Increases Insulin Resistance in Healthy Subjects." https://www.ncbi.nlm.nih.gov/pubmed/21036373

109 *Scientific Reports.* "A Low-Salt Diet Increases the Expression of Renal Sirtuin 1 Through Activation of the Ghrelin Receptor in Rats." https://www.nature.com/articles/srep32787

110 *McGill University–Science Daily.* "A New Role for Sodium in the Brain." https://www.sciencedaily.com/releases/2013/08/130820113931.htm

111 *Annals of Indian Academy of Neurology.* "The Effect of Curcumin (Turmeric) on Alzheimer's Disease." https://www.ncbi.nlm.nih.gov/pmc/articles/PMC2781139/

112 *European Journal of Nutrition.* "New Mechanisms and the Anti-Inflammatory Role of Curcumin in Obesity and Obesity-Related Metabolic Diseases." https://www.ncbi.nlm.nih.gov/pubmed/21442412

113 *Journal of Ethnopharmacology.* "Behavioral, Neurochemical and Neuroendocrine Effects of the Ethanolic Extract from *Curcuma longa l.* in the Mouse Forced Swimming Test." https://pubmed.ncbi.nlm.nih.gov/17134862/

114 *Appalachian State University.* "The Effects of Aerobic Exercise Timing on Sleep Architecture." https://libres.uncg.edu/ir/asu/listing.aspx?id=8000

115 *Salk News.* "Timing is Everything, To Our Genes." https://www.salk.edu/news-release/timing-everything-genes/

116 *British Journal of Nutrition, The.* "Nutrition and the Circadian System." https://www.ncbi.nlm.nih.gov/pmc/articles/PMC4930144/

117 *Cell Metabolism.* "A Smartphone App Reveals Erratic Diurnal Eating Patterns in Humans That Can Be Modulated for Health Benefits." https://www.cell.com/cell-metabolism/pdfExtended/S1550-4131(15)00462-3

118 *Obesity.* "Flipping the Metabolic Switch: Understanding and Applying Health Benefits of Fasting." https://www.ncbi.nlm.nih.gov/pmc/articles/PMC5783752/#!po=19.9115

119 *Journal of Applied Physiology.* "Effect of Intermittent Fasting and Refeeding on Insulin Action in Healthy Men." https://www.ncbi.nlm.nih.gov/pubmed/16051710

120 *Endocrinology.* "Intermittent Fasting Promotes Fat Loss with Lean Mass Retention, Increased Hypothalamic Norepinephrine Content, and Increased Neuropeptide Y Gene Expression in Diet-Induced Obese Male Mice." https://www.ncbi.nlm.nih.gov/pubmed/26653760

121 *Annals of Nutrition and Metabolism.* "Interleukin-6, C-Reactive Protein and Biochemical Parameters During Prolonged Intermittent Fasting." https://pubmed.ncbi.nlm.nih.gov/17374948/

122 *American Journal of Clinical Nutrition, The.* "Coffee Stimulation of Cholecystokinin Release and Gallbladder Contraction in Humans." https://www.ncbi.nlm.nih.gov/pubmed/2393014

123 *Biochemical Pharmacology.* "Anti-Diabetic and Anti-Lipidemic Effects of Chlorogenic Acid Are Mediated by AMPK Activation." https://www.ncbi.nlm.nih.gov/pubmed/23416115

RECIPE SECTION

1 *Obesity.* "Neural Responses to Visual Food Stimuli After a Normal Vs. Higher Protein Breakfast in Breakfast-Skipping Teens: A Pilot fMRI Study." https://pubmed.ncbi.nlm.nih.gov/21546927/

2 *Nutrients.* "The Relationship Between Vegetable Intake and Weight Outcomes: A Systematic Review of Cohort Studies." https://www.ncbi.nlm.nih.gov/pmc/articles/PMC6266069/

3 *International Journal of Molecular and Cellular Medicine.* "Differential Biological Behavior of Fibroblasts and Endothelial Cells Under Aloe Vera Gel Culturing." https://pubmed.ncbi.nlm.nih.gov/33274186/

4 *Mediators of Inflammation.* "Antiinflammatory and Immunomodulating Properties of Fungal Metabolites." https://www.ncbi.nlm.nih.gov/pmc/articles/PMC1160565/

5 *Pharmacology, Biochemistry, and Behavior.* "Extract of *Ganoderma lucidum* Potentiates Pentobarbital-Induced Sleep via a GABAergic Mechanism." https://www.sciencedirect.com/science/article/pii/S009130570700086X

6 *Neurology.* "Dehydration Confounds the Assessment of Brain Atrophy." https://n.neurology.org/content/64/3/548

7 *Journal of Physiology and Biochemistry.* "Dietary Fructooligosaccharides and Potential Benefits on Health." https://pubmed.ncbi.nlm.nih.gov/20119826/

8 *Current Opinion in Clinical Nutrition and Metabolic Care.* "L-Glycine: A Novel Antiinflammatory, Immunomodulatory, and Cytoprotective Agent." https://pubmed.ncbi.nlm.nih.gov/12589194/

9 *International Journal of Obesity.* "Gut Microbiome Diversity and High-Fiber Intake are Related to Lower Long-Term Weight Gain" https://www.nature.com/articles/ijo201766.

10 *PLoS One.* "Lactobacillus is Associated with Gut Microbial Changes and Reduction in Obesity." https://pubmed.ncbi.nlm.nih.gov/23555678/

11 *Journal of Nutrition, The.* "Cruciferous Vegetables Have Variable Effects on Biomarkers of Systemic Inflammation in a Randomized Controlled Trial in Healthy Young Adults." https://www.ncbi.nlm.nih.gov/pmc/articles/PMC4195422/

12 *British Journal of Nutrition, The.* "A Double-Blind, Placebo-Controlled, Cross-Over Study to Establish the Bifidogenic Effect of a Very-Long-Chain Inulin Extracted from Globe Artichoke in Healthy Human Subjects." https://pubmed.ncbi.nlm.nih.gov/20591206/

13 *American Journal of Clinical Nutrition, The.* "Insulin-Sensitizing Effects of Dietary Resistant Starch and Effects on Skeletal Muscle and Adipose Tissue Metabolism." https://www.ncbi.nlm.nih.gov/pubmed/16155268

14 *Journal of the American Dietetic Association.* "Chickpeas May Influence Fatty Acid and Fiber Intake in an Ad Libitum Diet, Leading to Small Improvements in Serum Lipid Profile and Glycemic Control." https://www.ncbi.nlm.nih.gov/pubmed/18502235

15 *Bioscience, Biotechnology & Biochemistry.* "Vinegar Intake Reduces Body Weight, Body Fat Mass, and Serum Triglyceride Levels in Obese Japanese Subjects." https://academic.oup.com/bbb/article/73/8/1837/5947518

16 *Food Science and Technology Research.* "Effects of Miso (Fermented Soybean Paste) Intake on Glycemic Index of Cooked Polished Rice." https://www.jstage.jst.go.jp/article/fstr/16/3/16_3_247/_pdf/-char/en

Recipe Index

Index

Note: Page numbers in **bold** indicate recipes

About the Author

Shawn Stevenson is a bestselling author and creator of the *Model Health Show*, featured as the #1 Health podcast in the U.S. with millions of listener downloads each year. A graduate of the University of Missouri–St. Louis, Shawn studied business, biology, and nutritional science, and went on to be the founder of Advanced Integrative Health Alliance, a company that provides wellness services for individuals and organizations worldwide. Shawn has been featured in *Forbes, Fast Company, Muscle & Fitness*, ABC News, ESPN, and many other major media outlets. He is also a frequent keynote speaker for numerous organizations, universities, and conferences.